Dermatology

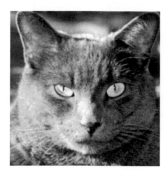

for the Small Animal Practitioner

by Ralf S. Mueller,
Dr. med.vet.,
MACVSc, DipACVD, FACVSc

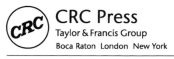

CRC Press
Taylor & Francis Group
Boca Raton London New York

CRC Press is an imprint of the
Taylor & Francis Group, an **informa** business

Dedication

To my wife, partner, and best friend, Sonya Bettenay, whose continued love, support, and feedback has helped me tremendously over the years personally and professionally. Without her this book would not have been possible.

To my parents, Irmi and Sigi, who encouraged and supported me when I left Germany to learn more about veterinary dermatology and who years later looked after the children to give me time to write this book.

To my children, Anya and Florian, whose interest and persistence in learning are a constant source of amazement and inspiration to me.

To my mentors, Peter Ihrke and Tony Stannard, and to all the colleagues whose support allowed me to develop the knowledge and experience that I hope will make this book useful in small animal practice. Specific thanks to Drs. Carol Foil, Gail Kunkle, Kerrie Lay, Helen Power, David Robson, and Linda Vogelnest, and the editorial team with Cindy Roantree, Susan Hunsberger, and Ray Lukens for their input and to Drs. Sonya Bettenay, Peter Ihrke, Thierry Olivry, Wayne Rosenkrantz, and Michael Shipstone for providing some of the pictures.

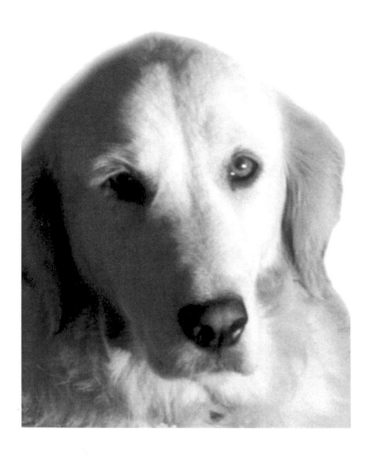

Preface

Dear Colleagues,

Veterinary dermatology plays an important role in small animal practice. Skin problems are the most frequent presenting complaint in many practices but due to their often chronic nature may cause frustration for veterinarians, clients, and patients alike.

This book is a practical introduction to veterinary dermatology for the busy small animal practitioner. It will help you to diagnose and manage skin diseases seen every day in your practice and allow you to perform a solid workup in patients with rare or complicated skin diseases that may require further reading, referral to, or advice from a veterinary dermatologist.

Most of all, I hope it **will allow you to enjoy your dermatology cases, provide good service, and improve the quality of life** in your patients.

Because your opinions and concerns are important in making this book most useful for the small animal practitioner, I would appreciate it if you would mail or email me any criticisms or suggestions for inclusion in future editions.

Warm regards,

Ralf S. Mueller,
Dr. med.vet., MACVSc, DipACVD, FACVSc

Department of Clinical Sciences
College of Veterinary Medicine and Biomedical Sciences
Colorado State University
Fort Collins, CO 80526, USA
Email: rmueller@vth.colostate.edu

Table of Contents

Section 1 "How To"

Section 2 The Approach to Common Dermatologic Presentations

Section 3 Treatments

Appendices 145

Recommended Readings

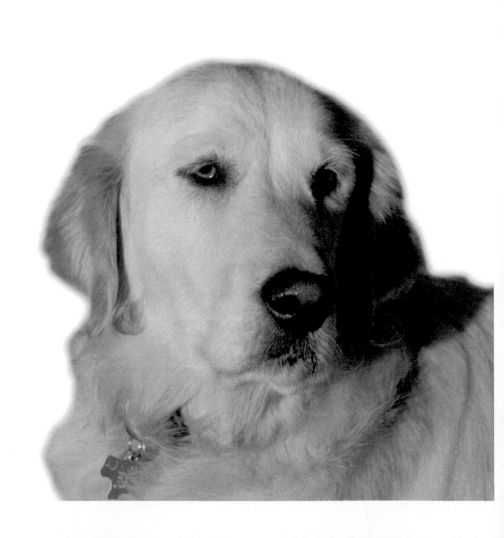

General Principles

The main goal of this book

is to provide a readily useable reference for veterinary dermatology that allows the thorough and logical workup of a patient seen for skin disease. It also provides therapeutic protocols for the most common dermatologic problems. There are three sections to this book. The first covers how to take a dermatologic history, interpret the results of this history in light of the clinical findings, and decide on and perform necessary tests. The second explains the approach to certain common dermatologic problems in small animal practice. The last summarizes therapeutic options for specific conditions.

Some Helpful Hints

Scattered throughout the text, you will find the following symbols to help you focus on what is really important:

✓   This is a routine feature of the subject discussed.

☛   We will use this selectively. This is a key point to understanding this particular topic.

✋   Stop. This does not look important, but it can really make a difference.

💣   Something serious will happen if you do not remember this, possibly resulting in the loss of both patient and client.

*   Drugs and Diseases marked with an asterisk and a colored screen in the tables in Sections 2 and 3, are potentially difficult and/or are dangerous. You may consider referral to a veterinary specialist or seek further advise from a colleague with more knowledge about the drug or disease.

Section 1

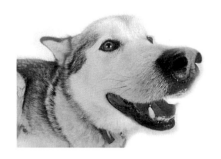

"How To"

In this section, I discuss key questions important in taking a dermatologic history and their implications, as well as specific dermatologic lesions and what they tell us. Furthermore, I introduce various tests important in veterinary dermatology, give their indications, explain necessary techniques in detail, and discuss the interpretation of the results.

Dermatologic History

Clinical signs for various skin diseases are very similar and the etiology of a patient's problem may not be apparent based solely on the findings of a clinical examination. A thorough history will typically provide clues in regard to the cause of the skin disorder and allow the veterinarian to prioritize time-consuming and frequently costly laboratory tests needed to confirm the diagnosis. I prefer my clients to fill out a questionnaire in the waiting room which we then review together during the consultation. This decreases the time needed to extract a good history from the owner, helps ensure a complete history independent of stress levels and time constraints, and allows the client to think about her or his pet's skin problem for a little while without unnecessarily delaying the appointment schedule. A sample of a dermatology questionnaire is enclosed in the Appendix. It is important to phrase questions appropriately, because many owners leave out pertinent facts either because they are not aware of their relevance or because they think these facts may not be well received by the veterinarian. Sometimes, it is necessary to ask the same question several times in different ways to obtain meaningful answers. I cannot overemphasize the importance of taking a good and efficient dermatologic history, which requires tremendous knowledge, experience, practice, and effective communication skills. To teach this is beyond the scope of this book. However, I do discuss some crucial questions and their implications in more detail.

Question: *What is the breed of the patient?*

Relevance

✓ Some breeds are predisposed to certain skin diseases and it may be worthwhile to keep a list of such breed predispositions in easy reach.

✓ A list of reported breed predisposition is given in the Appendix. But beware, breed predispositions may vary with geographic location!

Question: *How old was the patient when clinical signs were first recognized?*

Relevance

✓ Very young animals (puppies and kittens) are more commonly presented with congenital and hereditary defects, ectoparasites such as *Sarcoptes scabiei*, *Otodectes cynotis*, or *Demodex canis*, infections with bacteria (impetigo) or fungi (dermatophytosis) or, in dogs, canine juvenile sterile granulomatous dermatitis and lymphadenitis.

✓ Young adult dogs are more commonly affected by demodicosis, atopic dermatitis, and flea-bite hypersensitivity, as well as idiopathic seborrhea and follicular dysplasia.

✓ In middle age, hormonal diseases become a significant consideration, although allergies still occur in a significant number of animals, particularly in cats.

✓ Neoplastic diseases are more commonly seen in older animals.

Question: *How long has the disease been present and how did it progress?*

Relevance

✓ Acute onset of severe pruritus is frequently associated with scabies. Food adverse reaction may also have an explosive onset.

✓ If pruritus was the first initial sign and lesions occurred later, then atopy or food-adverse reaction are most likely. Pruritus with lesions that occur at approximately the same time may be due to a wide variety of causes.

✓ Chronic nonlesional pruritus is typically due to atopic dermatitis or food adverse reaction, possibly complicated by secondary infections. Scabies incognito may also cause nonlesional pruritus.

✓ If cutaneous signs have been present for years without the development of concurrent systemic signs, endocrine disorders are unlikely.

✓ Nonpruritic alopecia for years without systemic signs points towards alopecia and follicular dysplasias or hereditary alopecia.

✓ The presence of chronic wounds alone or associated with draining tracts necessitates the search for an infectious organism.

3

Diagnostic procedures: Scabies treatment trial, skin scrapings elimination diet, cytology, bacterial culture, fungal culture, biopsy.

Question: *Where on the body did the problem start?*

Relevance Tables 1-1 and 1-2 outline typically affected sites of certain diseases.

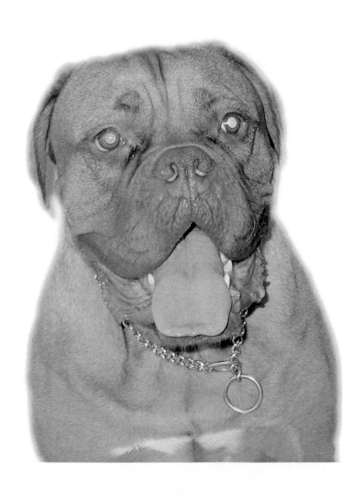

Table 1-1
Location of Lesions and/or Pruritus of
Various Canine Skin Diseases

LOCATION OF LESIONS AND/OR PRURITUS	COMMON UNDERLYING DISEASES
Otitis externa	Atopy, food adverse reaction, parasites, polyps. Secondary infections are common and can also occur with primary endocrine disease!
Pinnae	Atopy, food adverse reaction, scabies, vasculitis, pemphigus foliaceus
Head/face	Demodicosis, atopy, food adverse reaction, dermatophytosis, insect allergies, scabies, discoid lupus erythematosus, pemphigus foliaceus
Paws	Demodicosis, atopy, food adverse reaction, *Malassezia* dermatitis, pemphigus foliaceus, metabolic epidermal necrosis.
Claws	Bacterial or fungal infection, trauma, immune-mediated skin diseases.
Tail base	Flea-bite hypersensitivity

Table 1-2
Location of Lesions or Pruritus of
Various Feline Skin Diseases

LOCATION OF LESIONS AND/OR PRURITUS	COMMON UNDERLYING DISEASES
Otitis externa	Atopy, food adverse reaction, parasites, polyps. Secondary infections common!
Pinnae	*Notoedres cati,* vasculitis, pemphigus foliaceus
Head/face	Atopy, food adverse reaction, dermatophytosis, insect allergies, feline scabies, pemphigus foliaceus
Paws	Atopy, food adverse reaction, pemphigus foliaceus, trauma, plasmacytic pododermatitis
Claws	Bacterial infection, trauma, immune-mediated skin diseases
Tail base	Flea-bite hypersensitivity

Question: *Is the animal itchy?*

Relevance

✔ Pruritus is sometimes difficult to identify. Owners often do not consider licking, rubbing, or biting as clinical signs indicative of pruritus (we all have heard the story of the dog who is constantly licking its feet because "it is a very clean dog ..."). Several routine questions may be needed to identify pruritus in some patients: Are they licking or chewing their paws? Are they rubbing their faces? Do they scoot on their rear ends? Are they scratching their armpits?

✓ The presence of pruritus with skin lesions does not help much in discovering the etiology of the pruritus, given that many skin diseases cause pruritus. However, pruritus without lesions typically means either atopic dermatitis or food adverse reaction (possibly with secondary infections) or in rare instances scabies incognito.

✓ The perceived severity of pruritus may vary with the owner. Some owners deny the presence of pruritus despite the patient's frantic scratching in the consultation room. Others insist on severe pruritus in a patient with no evidence of self-trauma on clinical examination. Good communication skills and judgement are essential to form a realistic opinion for evaluation. If the pet's scratching wakes the owner up at night, the pruritus is severe irrespective of the presence of lesions.

✓ If itch preceeds the occurrence of lesions, atopic dermatitis, food adverse reaction, and scabies incognito must again be considered.

Diagnostic procedures: Trichogram in alopecic patients that are reportedly nonpruritic.

Question: *Is the disease seasonal?*

Relevance

✓ Insect bite hypersensitivities (caused most commonly by fleas, but mosquitoes or other insects can also be involved) frequently cause disease that worsens in summer. Whether clinical signs are absent or milder in the colder season depends on specific environmental conditions.

✓ Atopic dermatitis may also be seasonal in certain climates. In many temperate climates it may occur more noticeably in spring and summer if caused by tree and grass pollens or worsens in summer and autumn because of weed pollens. Warmer climates such as those found in tropical or subtropical regions usually have an extended pollen season. Hypersensitivities to house dust mites are often nonseasonal, but may be seasonally worse in winter in some areas and patients.

✓ Seasonal noninflammatory alopecia and hyperpigmentation may be due to cyclic follicular dysplasia.

Diagnostic procedures: Insect bite trial, intradermal skin testing, serum testing for allergen-specific IgE, biopsy, keeping the animal inside to evaluate for mosquito-bite hypersensitivity.

Question: *Are there other clinical signs such as sneezing, coughing, or diarrhea?*

Relevance

✓ Sneezing, coughing, wheezing, and conjunctivitis may be seen concurrently with atopic dermatitis and caused by airborne allergies.

✓ Diarrhea may be associated with food adverse reaction.

✓ Polydipsia and polyuria are common with iatrogenic and idiopathic hyperadrenocorticism.

✓ Systemic mycoses frequently present with concurrent anorexia, lethargy, and with gastrointestinal or respiratory symptoms.

Diagnostic procedures: Cytology of nasal exudate or conjunctiva, elimination diet, urine cortisol/creatinine ratio, low dose dexamethasone suppression test, and adrenocorticotropic hormone (ACTH)-stimulation test.

Question: *What is fed to the animal? Was a special diet used in the past? What was it and how long was it fed exclusively?*

Relevance

✓ Knowing the diet will allow the clinician to determine possible nutritional deficiencies.

✓ It will also help in formulating an elimination diet if indicated (p. 46).

✓ If a diet was fed in the past and it was not a true elimination diet (was not fed exclusively or not fed for an appropriate length of time) it may need to be repeated.

🔦 Contrary to the common belief, food adverse reactions typically do not occur immediately after a change in feeding habits. Most animals with food adverse reactions have been consuming the offending diet for years before showing clinical signs.

✋ Remember to ask about treats and supplements, which are often forgotten, when food is discussed with the client.

7

Question: *Are there other animals in the household? Do they show cutaneous symptoms?*

Relevance

✔ If other animals in the household are similarly affected, contagious disease such as dermatophytosis or scabies is more likely.

🖐 Other animals may serve as a reservoir for ectoparasites without showing clinical signs.

Diagnostic procedures: If indicated, insect control trial, fungal cultures, or scabies treatment trials should include all animals in the household to identify and/or treat possible carrier animals to allow successful long-term remission for the patient.

Question: *Does any person in the household have skin disease?*

Relevance

✔ Two zoonoses of major concern in veterinary dermatology are scabies and dermatophytosis (ringworm). However, even if owners are not affected, these diseases cannot be ruled out.

✔ Canine scabies affecting humans occurs as an itchy papular rash in contact areas, such as arms and legs, starting days to weeks after onset of pruritus in the pet.

✔ Dermatophytosis is often characterized by scaling and erythema and may not be particularly pruritic, but occasionally can present as severely inflammatory and pruritic skin disease. Dermatophytosis may sometimes be misdiagnosed as eczema in humans.

✔ Sporotrichosis and other mycoses have zoonotic potential and may occasionally cause disease in humans.

✔ Don't forget that the skin disease of the owner may also be completely unrelated to the animal's skin disease.

Diagnostic procedures: Wood's light, skin scrapings, fungal culture, scabies trial treatment. In severe forms of suspected dermatophytosis, a biopsy and special fungal stains may prove useful for obtaining a quick diagnosis.

Question: *Was the disease treated before? If so, which drugs were used and how successful was treatment?*

Relevance Response to previous therapy can be of tremendous help in establishing or ruling out underlying causes for the skin disease.

✔ Initial response to recent glucocorticoid administration may not be helpful because many skin diseases improve for a short period with this symptomatic, nonspecific treatment.

✔ Repeated response to low-dose glucocorticoid therapy suggests hypersensitivities (possibly complicated by *Malassezia* dermatitis caused by *Malassezia pachydermatis*).

✔ Repeated response to antibiotics and glucocorticoids in combination is of little help.

✔ Repeated partial or total response to antibiotics indicates a pyoderma usually secondary to either atopic dermatitis, food adverse reaction, hormonal disease, or another less common disorder that is suppressing the skin's immune system. In addition to antibacterial treatment, the underlying problem needs to be identified and treated to prevent recurrences.

✋ Ask specifically how much the pet improved while receiving medication because many owners tend to judge a treatment as not helpful if it did not cure the disease.

Question: *What is currently used to control fleas?*

Relevance

✔ Flea-bite hypersensitivity is the most common hypersensitivity and an extremely common skin disease in most small animal practices. If flea-bite hypersensitivity is suspected, a flea control trial should be commenced.

✔ Details of the flea control for all animals in the household are important because in a severely allergic animal, clinical signs can be caused by a very small number of flea bites. Inconsistent or ineffective flea control can be discovered only through detailed questioning.

✋ Many owners take questions about their flea control as an insult to their own cleanliness and hygiene. Good communication skills are a great help. I own a flea-allergic dog and routinely mention her as an example, which breaks the ice and increases the client's willingness to listen and follow my instructions.

Question: *When was the last medication given?*

Relevance

✔ Recent administration of medication may affect the clinical presentation.

✓ It may also affect various indicated diagnostic tests that may need to be postponed.

✓ Long-term glucocorticoid therapy will affect the results of allergy tests – both intradermal skin testing and serum testing for allergen-specific IgE. It will also affect histopathologic findings and the results of many blood tests.

✓ Antihistamines and short-term systemic and topical glucocorticoids (i.e., < 4 weeks) may influence intradermal skin testing.

✓ Some antibiotics, such as trimethoprim-sulfonamide combinations, will affect blood concentrations of thyroxin. Others such as cephalosporins may affect the glucose readings of some urine test strips.

✓ Remember to ask specific questions regarding heartworm prevention, vitamin supplements, or deworming which are also forms of pharmacotherapy.

Question: *Does the animal get better with a change of environment (a weekend away or a day at the in-laws for example)?*

Relevance

✓ The animal's improvement in another environment indicates involvement of an environmental allergen (airborne or contact) or irritant.

✓ Lack of improvement does not rule out these allergies, in that airborne and contact allergens may be the same in different locations (house dust mites are found almost anywhere in the world).

Dermatologic Examination

A good dermatologic examination requires adequate lighting, a systematic and thorough approach, and should always include a general physical examination. Observation from a distance should be followed by close inspection of skin and mucous membranes. I start at the head, look at the lips, mouth, ears, run my hands through the coat of the trunk, lift up the tail to inspect the peri-anal area, and then examine the legs and feet with pads and claws. Next, the patient is rolled on his back – reluctant small pets are made to sit up in the lap of the owner; with larger dogs the front paws are lifted up for a short moment, which gives me the opportunity to examine the animal's ventral aspects from the axillae to the groin.

General Observation

Localized or Generalized Problem

✓ Localized problems may be due to infectious organisms that gained entry at a certain site and spread only locally such as atypical mycobacterial or fungal infections.

✓ Neoplastic disease is commonly localized, at least initially.

✓ Generalized disorders are more commonly due to hypersensitivities or systemic conditions such as endocrine disorders and immune-mediated or metabolic skin diseases.

Symmetry

✓ Bilaterally symmetric lesions are typically caused by internal disease such as hypothyroidism, hyperadrenocorticism, or pemphigus foliaceus. Allergies may also present with bilaterally symmetric symptoms.

✓ Asymmetric lesions more commonly have external causes such as ectoparasites (e.g., demodicosis) or fungi (e.g., dermatophytosis).

Haircoat Quality, Color, and Shine

✓ Is the haircoat dull or shiny? A dull haircoat may be due to metabolic or hormonal diseases, nutritional deficiencies, or chronic skin disease.

✓ Are there color abnormalities or changes and if so, did they occur before or concurrent with the onset of skin disease or as a consequence of the disease. Hair color changes may be associated with hormonal disease or follicular dysplasia.

✓ Changes in the hair quality (either to a coarse coat or to a fine puppy coat) may again point to hormonal disease or follicular dysplasia.

Close inspection of the skin and mucous membranes follows the general observation. Pay special attention to any individual lesions. Primary lesions are initial eruptions that are caused directly by the underlying disease process. Secondary lesions evolve from primary lesions or are caused by the patient (self-trauma) or environment (medications). It is important that the clinician be able both to differentiate between primary and secondary lesions and to understand the underlying pathomechanism because this helps in the formulation of a relevant list of differential diagnoses. I next discuss the individual lesions and their implications and give the most common differential diagnoses for each lesion.

Primary Lesions
Macule

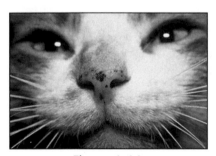

Figure 1-1A
Macule

Definition: A focal, circumscribed, nonpalpable change in color <1 cm (when it is larger, it is termed a patch). Pathogenesis: Pigmentation change due to decreased or increased melanin production, erythema due to inflammation or local hemorrhage caused by trauma or vasculitis.

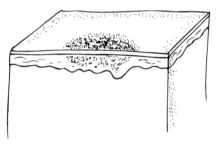

Figure 1-1B
Macule

Differential diagnoses-depigmentation: Vitiligo, discoid lupus erythematosus, uveodermatologic syndrome, mucocutaneous pyoderma.
Differential diagnoses-hyperpigmentation: Lentigo, hormonal diseases or post-inflammatory with a multitude of possible underlying causes lentigo. **Differential diagnosis-erythema:** Inflammation due to a variety of underlying diseases or hemorrhage due to vasculopathies or coagulopathies.

Papule

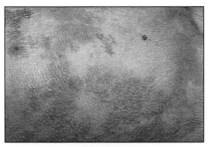

Figure 1-2A
Papule

Definition: A solid elevation of up to 1 cm in diameter. Larger lesions are called plaques. Pathogenesis: Influx of inflammatory cells into the dermis, focal epidermal hyperplasia, early neoplastic lesions.

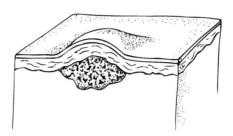

Figure 1-2B
Papule

Differential diagnoses: Bacterial folliculitis, demodicosis, fungal folliculitis, flea-bite and mosquito-bite hypersensitivity, scabies, contact allergy, autoimmune skin disease, drug eruption.

Pustule

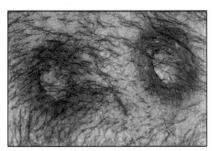

Figure 1-3A
Pustule

Definition: A small circumscribed area within the epidermis filled with pus. Pathogenesis: Most pustules are filled with neutrophils, but eosinophilic pustules may also be seen. Aspiration cytology and biopsy are indicated. (Courtesy of Dr. Thierry Olivry.)

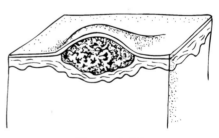

Figure 1-3B
Pustule

Differential diagnoses-neutrophils: Bacterial infection, fungal infection, autoimmune skin disease.
Differential diagnoses-eosinophils: Insect or contact hypersensitivity, parasites, immune-mediated skin disease

Vesicle

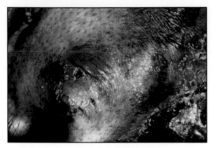

Figure 1-4A
Vesicle

Definition: A small circumscribed area within or below the epidermis filled with clear fluid. Larger vesicles are called bullae. Vesicles are very fragile and thus transient. Pathogenesis: Spongiosis and extra-cellular fluid collection due to inflammation and loss of cohesion. (Courtesy of Dr. Thierry Olivry)

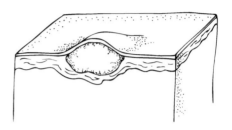

Figure 1-4B
Vesicle

Differential diagnoses: Immune-mediated and congenital skin diseases, viral diseases, or irritant dermatitis.

Wheal

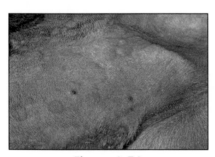

Figure 1-5A
Wheal

Definition: A sharply circumscribed, raised, edematous lesion that appears and disappears within minutes to hours. Pathogenesis: Subcutaneous edema.

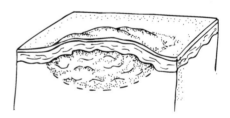

Figure 1-5B
Wheal

Differential diagnoses: Urticaria, insect bites, other hypersensitivities, drug eruption.

Nodule

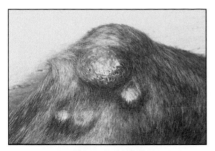

Figure 1-6A
Nodule

Definition: A circumscribed, solid elevation more than 1 cm in diameter that extends into deeper layers of the skin. Pathogenesis: Massive infiltration of inflammatory or neoplastic cells into the dermis and subcutis or deposition of fibrin and crystalline material.

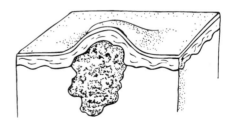

Figure 1-6B
Nodule

Differential diagnoses: Sterile granulomatous diseases, bacterial or fungal infections, neoplastic diseases, calcinosis cutis

Tumor

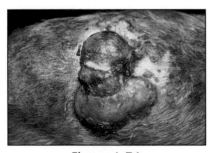

Figure 1-7A
Tumor

Definition: A large mass involving skin or subcutaneous tissue. Pathogenesis: Massive influx of inflammatory or neoplastic cells.

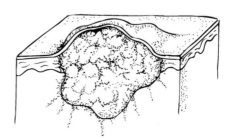

Figure 1-7B
Tumor

Differential diagnoses: Sterile granulomatous diseases, bacterial or fungal infections, neoplastic diseases.

Primary or Secondary Lesions

Alopecia

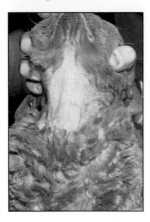

Figure 1-8
Alopecia

Definition: Partial to complete loss of hair. Pathogenesis: Self-trauma, damage to the hair or hair follicle due to dysplasia, inflammation and/or infection, lack of hair regrowth often due to hormonal disease.

Differential diagnoses: Primary lesion in follicular dysplasias, endocrine disorders, telogen effluvium, anagen defluxion. Secondary lesion in pruritic skin diseases, bacterial or fungal folliculitis, demodicosis.

Scale

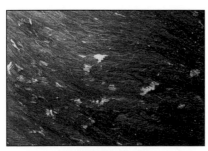

Figure 1-9A
Scale

Definition: An accumulation of loose fragments of the horny layer of the skin. Pathogenesis: Increased production of keratinocytes (often associated with abnormalities of the keratinization process) or increased retention of corneocytes.

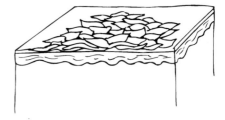

Figure 1-9B
Scale

Differential diagnoses: Primary lesion in follicular dysplasias, idiopathic seborrheas and ichthyosis. Secondary lesion in diseases associated with chronic skin inflammation.

Crust

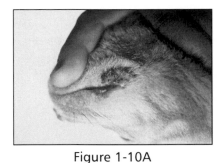

Figure 1-10A
Crust

Definition: Adherence of dried exudate, serum, pus, blood, scales, or medications to the skin surface.

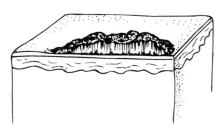

Figure 1-10B
Crust

Differential diagnoses: Primary lesion in idiopathic seborrhea, zinc-responsive dermatitis, metabolic epidermal necrosis. Secondary lesion in a variety of skin diseases.

Follicular Cast

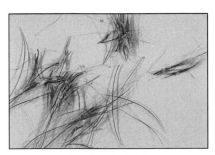

Figure 1-11A
Follicular cast

Definition: An accumulation of keratin and follicular material to the hair shaft.

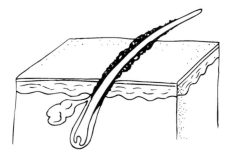

Figure 1-11B
Follicular cast

Differential diagnoses: Primary lesion in vitamin A-responsive dermatosis, idiopathic seborrhea, and sebaceous adenitis. Secondary lesion in dermatophytosis and demodicosis.

Pigmentary Abnormalities

Hyperpigmentation

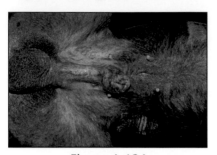

Figure 1-12A
Hyperpigmentation

Definition: Increased epidermal and/or dermal melanin. Pathogenesis: Increased production, size, or melanization of melanosomes or increased number of melanosomes due to a variety of intrinsic or extrinsic factors. Most common cause: Chronic inflammation

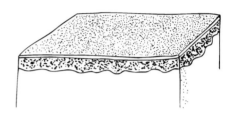

Figure 1-12B
Hyperpigmentation

Differential diagnoses: Primary lesion in endocrine dermatoses, secondary postinflammatory change due to a variety of skin diseases.

Comedo

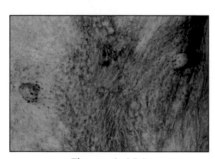

Figure 1-13A
Comedones

Definition: A dilated hair follicle filled with corneocytes and sebaceous material. Pathogenesis: Primary keratinization defects or hyperkeratosis due to hormonal abnormalities or inflammation.

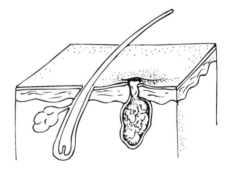

Figure 1-13B
Comedones

Differential diagnoses: Primary lesion in feline acne, some idiopathic seborrheas, Schnauzer comedo syndrome, endocrine diseases. Secondary lesion in demodicosis, and less commonly dermatophytosis.

Secondary Lesions

Epidermal Collarette

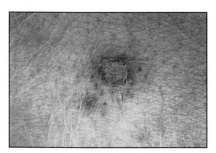

Figure 1-14A
Epidermal collarette

Definition: Scale of loose keratin flakes or "peeling" keratin arranged in a circle. Pathogenesis: Remnant of a pustule or vesicle after the top part (the "roof") has been lost, or caused by a point source of inflammation, such as a papule.

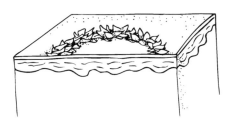

Figure 1-14B
Epidermal collarette

Differential diagnoses: Most likely bacterial infection, less commonly fungal infection, immune-mediated skin disease, insect-bite reaction, or contact hypersensitivity.

Erosion

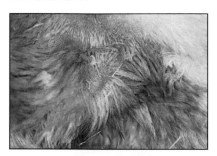

Figure 1-15A
Erosion

Definition: A shallow epidermal defect that does not penetrate the basal membrane. Pathogenesis: Trauma or inflammation leads to rapid death and/or loss of keratinocytes

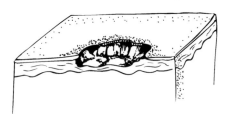

Figure 1-15B
Erosion

Differential diagnoses: Various skin diseases associated with self trauma such as infections or allergies.

Ulcer

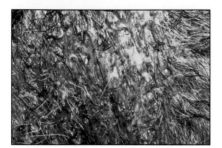

Figure 1-16A
Ulcer

Definition: Focal loss of epidermis with exposure of underlying dermis
Pathogenesis: Severe trauma and/or deep and severe inflammation

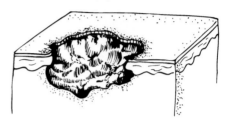

Figure 1-16B
Ulcer

Differential diagnoses: Various skin diseases associated with trauma such as infections and allergies, also immune-mediated diseases.

Lichenification

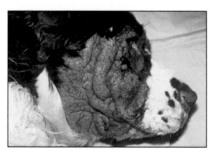

Figure 1-17A
Lichenification

Definition: Thickening and hardening of skin characterized by exaggerated superficial skin markings.
Pathogenesis: Chronic trauma such as friction or rubbing.

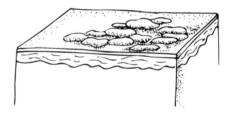

Figure 1-17B
Lichenification

Differential diagnoses: All chronic and pruritic skin diseases.

Specific Tests in Small Animal Dermatology

Cytology

Indications

Any pruritic, scaly, odoriferous, or alopecic animal should be evaluated for evidence of bacterial or fungal infection. Thus, cytology is indicated for almost all patients presented with skin disease. Skin scrapings, aspirations, impressions, ear swabs and tape preparations are different techniques to obtain cytologic samples.

✓ A superficial skin scraping is used in areas such as the interdigital skin where impression smears may be difficult to obtain. It is also used when the skin is normal, slightly moist, or greasy.

✓ An aspirated sample is useful in the evaluation of pustule content and intracutaneous or subcutaneous nodules.

✓ An impression smear is used when moist or oily skin with oozing or discharging lesions is evaluated.

✓ Ear swabs are used to evaluate ear canals.

✓ Dry scaly skin maybe evaluated by tape preparations. This technique is also frequently used in the interdigital area where impression smears may be difficult to obtain.

Technique

1. Skin scraping for cytology

✓ Affected skin is exposed and the surface of the skin scraped very gently and superficially with a scalpel blade in the direction of hair growth.

✓ The debris collected on the blade is applied to a slide and spread with the blade in a "buttering the bread" motion (Figure 1-18).

2. Aspiration of nodules

✓ Aspiration from nodules or abscesses is undertaken with a 12-ml syringe and a 22-ga needle.

✓ The nodule is firmly grasped and the needle is then inserted (Figure 1-19), aspirated several times (up to the 10-ml mark if possible), the pressure released, and the syringe with needle still attached is withdrawn.

✓ It is important to release the pressure before withdrawal of the needle or else the aspirate can be sucked back into the barrel of the syringe – from which it may not be retrieved.

✓ The needle is detached, the plunger pulled back, and the needle reattached.

✓ Cells are then blown onto a slide. The smear is air dried.

3. Impression Smears

✓ Cotton swabs are used to obtain samples from ear canals by inserting them into the canal, rotating, and withdrawing them. They are then rolled gently onto a slide. I hold ear slides uniformly on the left side with my left hand, the cotton swab from the left ear is rolled onto the mid-section of the slide and the cotton swab from the right ear onto the right third of the same slide.

✓ In patients with dry skin, a cotton swap may be moistened with saline solution and rubbed on the surface of affected skin before it is rolled onto a slide.

✓ In patients with moist or greasy skin, the slide can be rubbed or impressed directly onto affected skin (Figure 1-20).

4. Tape Preparation

✓ A direct impression technique uses clear sticky tape to collect debris from the surface of the skin. Although quick, this method does take practice to establish what is "normal."

✓ The tape is pressed sticky side down onto the skin (Figure 1-21).

✓ Next, it is pressed (also sticky side down) onto a drop of methylene blue or the blue stain of DiffQuick on a slide (Figure 1-22).

✓ The tape serves as a cover slip: the sample can be evaluated even under oil immersion (with a small droplet of oil placed directly on top of the tape).

✓ This technique is especially useful for *Malassezia* evaluation. Other items of interest that can be identified include inflammatory cells such as neutrophils (which may have passed through the epidermis in response to a superficial infection), nucleated epithelial cells (which are not normal and reflect a keratinization abnormality), cocci, rods, macrophages, short-bodied demodex mites, *Cheyletiella*, and occasionally *Sarcoptes* mites.

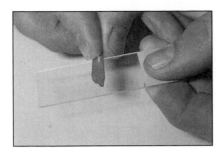

Figure 1-18
Debris collected with a superficial skin scraping is spread onto a slide with a "butter the bread" motion.

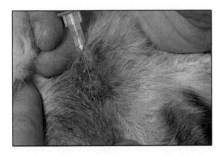

Figure 1-19
Aspiration of a small nodule.

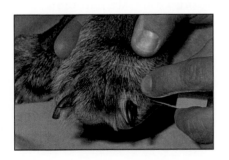

Figure 1-20
Impression smears are obtained by gently pressing a slide onto affected skin.

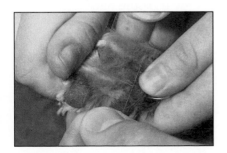

Figure 1-21
The tape is pressed sticky-side down onto affected skin.

Stain

✓ A modified Wright's stain (e.g., DiffQuick) can be used to stain the air-dried slides. It is much faster and easier than Gram's stain and sufficient to evaluate nearly all skin cytology samples. But Gram's stain is also suitable.

Interpretation

✓ Yeast organisms are most often M. *pachydermatis* (Figure 1-23), although *Candida* spp. may occasionally be involved.

✓ Cocci are most often *Staphylococcus intermedius* (Figure 1-24). *S. aureus* or *Streptococci* may be found in some patients.

✓ Rod-shaped organisms are found mostly in the ear canal and are most often *Pseudomonas aeruginosa* or *Proteus mirabilis* (Figure 1-25).

☛ The number of organisms is important. Occasional cocci or yeast are probably not relevant. On the skin, I consider one or more yeast organisms per high-power field (HPF) relevant; cocci should be seen in high numbers. In the infected ear, yeast and cocci typically occur in high numbers; any rods present are abnormal. Don't mistake exogenous bacterial contaminants for infection.

✓ Inflammatory cells with intracellular organisms are pathognomonic for a clinically relevant infection (Figure 1-26).

✓ Eosinophils typically indicate allergic or parasitic skin disease.

💣 Neoplastic cells may be difficult to recognize so that the help of a clinical pathologist is typically needed. Even with high skill levels, neoplastic skin disease should not be diagnosed exclusively by cytology (with the exception of mast cell tumors); a biopsy should always confirm any suspicions raised clinically and cytologically.

✓ If mast cells are found cytologically (Figure 1-27), the diagnosis of mast cell tumor is confirmed, but complete surgical excision should still be confirmed by histopathology. In some patients with mast cell tumors, mast cell granules do not stain with routine DiffQuick and thus a negative cytologic result can not rule out mastocytosis.

✓ Acantholytic cells are keratinocytes that have lost their intercellular connections (desmosomes) and present as round cells with a purple cytoplasm and a central dark purple nucleus (Figure 1-28). These cells suggest pemphigus foliaceus or erythematosus but can also be seen on cytologic samples of severe pyodermas. A biopsy is indicated to confirm the diagnosis.

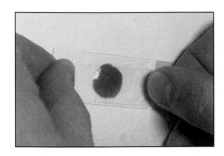

Figure 1-22
Tape is then pressed sticky-side down onto a drop of methylene blue on a slide.

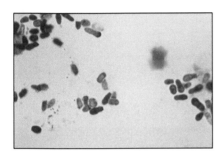

Figure 1-23
Malassezia pachydermatis on a tape preparation stained with blue stain of DiffQuick (original magnification x400).

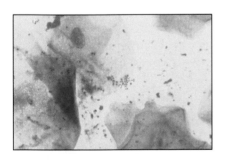

Figure 1-24
Cocci on an impression smear stained with DiffQuick (original magnification x1000).

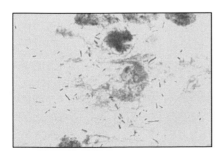

Figure 1-25
Rods on an impression smear obtained from otitis externa and stained with DiffQuick (original magnification x1000).

☞ Remember, that bacterial and yeast infections are usually secondary to other diseases, which need to be identified and treated to prevent recurrence of the infection.

☞ Cytologic re-evaluation at the end of antimicrobial therapy is crucial because organisms may change during treatment. For instance, a dog initially presented with bacterial infection may develop a yeast infection during successful antibacterial treatment, preventing clinical improvement and vice versa.

Treatment of bacterial infections and antifungal therapy are discussed in Section 3.

Superficial Skin Scrapings

Indications

Any pruritic or scaly dog and cat may be infested with *Cheyletiella* spp., *Otodectes cynotis, Scabies scabiei,* or *Notoedres-cati* and should be scraped.

Technique

✔ If scabies is suspected, preferred areas for scrapings are the elbows, hocks, and ventrum. Ear margins should be scraped thoroughly if any pruritus or scaling is observed in this area. Sometimes scaling is subtle and only becomes evident on close examination.

✔ Sites are gently clipped with #40 clipper blades. Mites may be difficult to find (especially canine scabies mites), so that the bigger the surface area scraped, the greater will be the chance of a positive skin scraping.

🖐 Several drops of mineral oil are applied directly to the clipped skin and distributed evenly in the area.

✔ The oil is scraped off with a #11 scalpel blade (Figure 1-29) and transferred to one or more glass slide(s). Scrape 10 to 15 times especially when canine scabies is suspected.

✔ A cover slip is used to allow rapid yet thorough evaluation of collected debris (Figure 1-30) and the slide(s) is (are) evaluated under low power (x40 or x100) systematically from the left upper corner to the right lower corner.

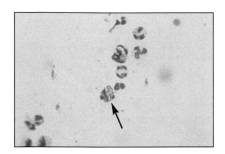

Figure 1-26
Neutrophils with intracellular cocci (arrow) pathognomonic for bacterial infection stained with DiffQuick (original magnification x1000).

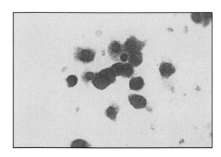

Figure 1-27
Mast cells on an aspirate from a feline mast cell tumor stained with DiffQuick (original magnification x1000).

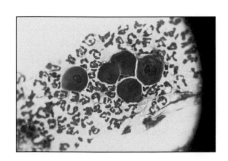

Figure 1-28
Acantholytic cells on an aspirate of an intact pustule from a dog with pemphigus foliaceus stained with DiffQuick (original magnification x1000).

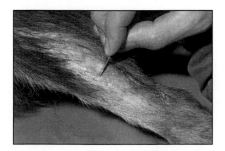

Figure 1-29
A scalpel blade is used to scrape applied oil off the affected and clipped skin.

Interpretation

A finding of one mite or egg of *Sarcoptes spp.*, *Notoedres cati*, *Cheyletiella spp.* or *Otodectes cynotis* (Figures 1-31, 1-32, and 1-33) is diagnostic for the cause of the skin disease. Negative scrapings do not rule out the presence of mites and clinical disease particularly in canine scabies. *Cheyletiella spp.* and *Otodectes cynotis* may also be missed by superficial skin scrapings. The next step would be a therapeutic trial (p. 49), possibly in conjunction with other diagnostic tests such as an elimination diet (p. 46) to evaluate other causes of pruritus.

Deep Skin Scrapings

Indication

Any dog or cat with possible demodicosis must be scraped. Thus, every alopecic patient and every patient with papules, pustules, crusting, and particularly interdigital pododermatitis must be scraped for the presence of demodicosis. Effective deep skin scrapings of paws may require sedation or general anesthesia.

Technique

🖐 Because *Demodex canis* and *felis* mites live deep in the hair follicle, it is useful to squeeze the skin as hard as the patient can tolerate before scraping in an attempt to push mites out from the depths of the follicles.

🔪 A blade covered with mineral oil should be used in the direction of hair growth until capillary bleeding is observed (Figure 1-34).

🖐 Feet and faces are hard to scrape, so that it may be worthwhile to scrape erythematous areas adjacent to papules and crusts interdigitally to maximize the yield and to minimize bleeding associated with scraping. Hair plucks may be useful for those areas, the plucked hair is placed in a drop of mineral oil on a slide, with a cover slip and evaluated microscopically for the presence of mites (p. 38).

✓ Negative scrapings or hair plucks of interdigital areas do not rule out pododemodicosis; a biopsy may be needed to confirm or rule out the diagnosis.

✓ Old English Sheepdogs, Scottish Terriers and especially Shar-peis may produce negative results on scrapings and may have to be biopsied for diagnosis. Although not documented, it is thought that these breeds have more tortuous and deeper hair follicles.

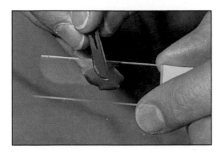

Figure 1-30
...and the oil and gathered debris are transferred to a slide.

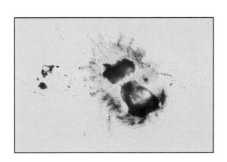

Figure 1-31
Sarcoptes scabiei mites and eggs obtained with a superficial skin scraping from a dog with scabies (original magnification x40).

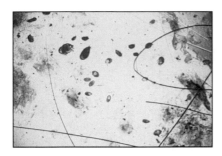

Figure 1-32
Cheyletiella parasitivorax (original magnification x40).

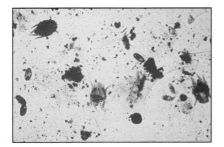

Figure 1-33
Otodectes cynotis mites and eggs (original magnification x40). (Courtesy of Dr. Peter Ihrke.)

✓ The finding of more than one mite should be considered diagnostic.

Interpretation

✓ It is important to assess the relative numbers of adults (both live and dead), larvae/nymphs and eggs (Figure 1-35) per low power field (LPF) and to record the site of scraping. During subsequent visits, assessment of response to therapy relies on the comparison of such numbers, so we routinely repeat scrapes at the same sites monthly when monitoring cases with demodicosis.

Treatment for demodicosis is outlined in Section 3.

Wood's Lamp Examination

Indication

Any dog or cat with possible Microsporum canis infection should be examined with a Wood's lamp. Any patient with alopecia, papules, pustules, and/or crusts may benefit from the procedure.

Technique

✓ The Wood's lamp should be warmed up for 5 minutes before use because the stability of the light's wavelength and intensity depends on temperature.

✓ The animal is examined under the lamp in a dark room.

☝ Hairs invaded by M. canis may show a yellow-green fluorescence. This fluorescence runs along the hair shafts (Figure 1-36) rather than fluorescing on discrete, individual, occasional scales, as may be seen in normal animals and humans.

✓ Some drugs, soaps, and bacteria such as Pseudomonas aeruginosa may also cause fluorescence but are usually not associated with hair shafts.

Interpretation

✓ In approximately 50% of all infections with M. canis, greenish fluorescence of tryptophan metabolites is seen under ultraviolet light at 253.7 nm.

✓ Positive fluorescence is diagnostic for dermatophytosis and by far the most common fluorescing dermatophyte in veterinary medicine is M. canis. Some other dermatophytes may show fluorescence, but these are not relevant in veterinary dermatology.

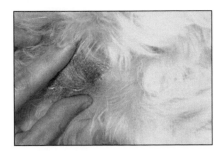

Figure 1-34

To evaluate a patient for demodicosis, scrapings must be deep, until capillary bleeding is observed. The skin should be squeezed to maximize the yield.

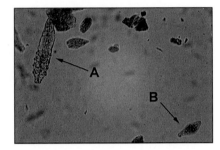

Figure 1-35

Demodex canis (A) mite and (B) egg (original magnification x100).

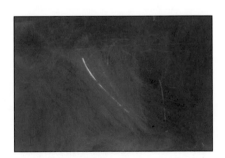

Figure 1-36

Green fluorescent hair shafts under Wood's lamp examination in a cat infected with M. *canis.*

☞ A lack of fluorescence does not rule out dermatophytosis. Fungal culture and/or biopsy are the next steps.

Treatment of dermatophytosis is outlined in Section 3.

Fungal Culture

Indication

A fungal culture may be indicated in any dog or cat with possible fungal infection and thus in any patient with alopecia, papules, pustules, and/or crusts.

Technique

✓ Hairs and scale from the edge of a lesion (preferably the ones fluorescing under the Wood's lamp) should be taken (Figure 1-37).

✓ If lesions are not well circumscribed or if asymptomatic carriers are suspected, I recommend the McKenzie tooth brush method. In this technique, the hair is brushed with a sterile toothbrush (any new tooth brush in a sealed package is sufficiently sterile mycologically). Scales and loose hairs caught in the tooth brush are gently imprinted onto the agar (Figure 1-38).

✓ Sabouraud's agar is the most common medium for fungal cultures. In practice dermatophyte test medium (DTM) is frequently used. DTM is essentially a Sabouraud agar with a color indicator and added ingredients to inhibit overgrowth with saprophytes and bacteria.

✋ After being innoculated, the culture jars should be incubated at between 25° and 30° C at 30% humidity, or in a warm dark corner with the lids not screwed down tightly.

✓ Cultures should be incubated for 2 to 3 weeks and must be evaluated daily.

Interpretation

☞ A pH change (and subsequent color change) that occurs as the colony grows indicates dermatophytes (Figure 1-39). These fungi use protein and produce alkaline metabolites which cause the pH and color change. It is imperative that the color change is observed coincidentally with the development of the colony. Color changes also occur in association with mature (i.e., large) saprophyte colonies. Saprophytes initially utilize carbohydrates. Once all carbohydrates have been used and the colony is already grown (Figure 1-40), they turn to the proteins and rapidly change the color and pH with the subsequent

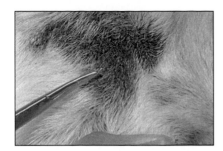

Figure 1-37
Hairs and scales from the edge of skin lesions are chosen for fungal culture.

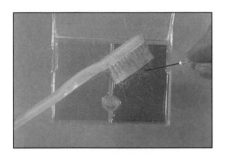

Figure 1-38
Contents of a tooth brush are transferred to a fungal culture medium after using the McKenzie toothbrush technique.

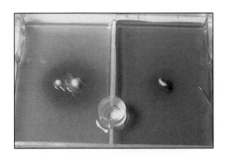

Figure 1-39
A dermatophyte culture changes the color of the dermatophyte test medium in early stages of growth.

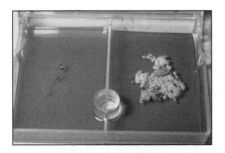

Figure 1-40
A large saprophyte colony prior to color change.

alkaline metabolites (Figure 1-41). It may be impossible to distinguish on gross appearance whether a mature colony with significant red pigmentation to the underlying and surrounding agar is a pathogenic or saprophytic fungus.

✓ Always check the colony microscopically for characteristic macroconidia. Clear sticky tape is impressed gently onto the culture (sticky side down), then laid onto a drop of methylene blue or the blue stain of DiffQuick (also sticky side down) on a microscope slide and evaluated under the microscope. The surface of the sticky tape acts as its own cover slip. If required, microscope oil can be placed directly onto the surface of the tape.

✓ *Microsporum canis* grows in a white, wooly colony with a yellowish reverse pigment (which maybe difficult to assess if grown on DTM). Abundant spindle-shaped macroconidia with knobs at the terminal ends and typically more than six internal compartments are seen microscopically (Figure 1-42).

🖐 M. *canis* is a zoophilic fungus and patients typically were infected by another animal or human. Humans and other animals in contact with the patient are at risk to develop the infection or may be asymptomatic carriers and need to be carefully evaluated and possibly treated as well.

✓ M. *gypseum* grows in a granular beige culture with yellowish reverse pigment and has thin-walled echinulate macroconidia with fewer than six internal compartments (Figure 1-43). M. *gypseum* is a geophilic fungus that is acquired by exposure to contaminated soil and thus has a limited zoonotic potential.

✓ Trichophyton mentagrophytes grow in colonies of variable texture and color that characteristically have a few cigar-shaped macroconidia and globous microconidia (Figure 1-44). Typical hosts for *T. mentagrophytes* are rodents and humans; infections are usually associated with exposure to these hosts or their immediate environment.

See Section 3 for treatment of dermatophytosis

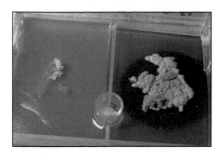

Figure 1-41
Saprophyte colony of Figure 1-40
24 hours later.

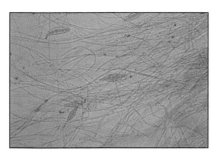

Figure 1-42
Hyphae and macroconidia of
Microsporum canis.

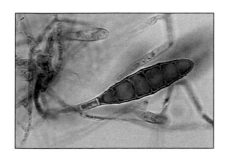

Figure 1-43
Hyphae and macroconidia of
Microsporum gypseum.

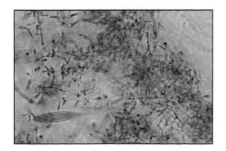

Figure 1-44
Hyphae and microconidia of *Trichophyton
mentagrophytes*.

Trichogram

Indication

Trichograms may be useful in any alopecic animal as well as in animals with suspected dermatophytosis and associated papules, pustules, or crusting.

Technique

✓ A forceps is used to forcefully pluck hairs from affected skin (Figure 1-45).

✓ The hairs are then placed onto a slide and evaluated under low power. I generally use mineral oil and a cover slip to prevent the hair sample from blowing all over the table rather than remaining under the microscope (Figure 1-46).

Interpretation

A trichogram is taken for several reasons:

✓ To determine how many hairs are in telogen (or resting) versus anagen (or growing) phase (in shedding or suspected endocrine problems). This requires practice! Anagen-phase bulbs are rounded, smooth, shiny, glistening and soft so the root may bend (Figure 1-47). Telogen bulbs are club- or spear-shaped with a rough surface (Figure 1-48). A sample with exclusively or mostly telogen hairs points to an endocrine disorder or follicular arrest.

✓ To determine if a cat or dog creates hair loss by licking or rubbing, or if the hair falls out for another reason. If the animal is pruritic and licks the hair off, the tips of the hairs are broken off (Figure 1-49). Any trauma to the hair shaft, such as occurs in dermatophytosis or anagen defluxion, may also cause hair with broken ends. If the hair falls out for other reasons, the tips are tapered (Figure 1-50).

✓ Trichograms are used routinely in human dermatology to evaluate alopecias, but their usefulness in veterinary dermatology has not been explored in any great detail and is hampered by the marked variations in breed characteristics.

🔑 A trichogram is most useful to determine if bald cats that present with a history of "nonpruritic" alopecia are really so-called "closet lickers" or "hidden groomers" (in which case the hair-shaft ends will be fractured) or if the hair falls out due to telogen effluvium or, very rarely, for hormonal reasons.

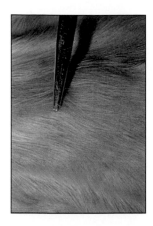

Figure 1-45
A forceps is used to pull hairs from affected skin for a trichogram.

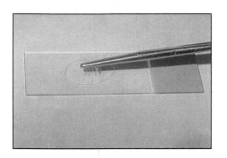

Figure 1-46
The hairs are placed in oil onto a slide under a cover slip.

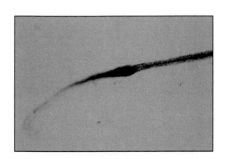

Figure 1-47
Anagen bulbs in a trichogram of a normal dog (original magnification x100).

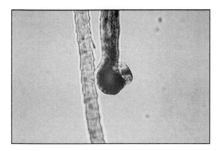

Figure 1-48
Telogen bulb in a trichogram of a dog with hyperadrenocorticism (original magnification x100).

⊶ Trichograms may also be used to diagnose canine demodicosis. If mites are found microscopically, the diagnosis is confirmed. However, if no mites are present, demodicosis cannot be ruled out!

⊶ Trichograms can also help to diagnose color-diluent alopecia. In this disease the melanin in the hair shaft is present in big clumps rather than finely dispersed as in normal pigmented hair.

Biopsy

Indication

✓ Any skin that appears unusual to the clinician should be biopsied.

✓ A biopsy should also be considered if lesions fail to respond to appropriate empiric therapy.

✓ Nodules are possibly neoplastic and should be biopsied.

✓ The presence of any suspected disease for which treatment is expensive and/or life-threatening should be confirmed histopathologically.

✓ One of the major reasons to perform a skin biopsy is to rule out other diagnoses ("I think this is an allergy but... "). In such a situation, the biopsy report of "chronic hyperplastic dermatitis with mononuclear perivascular infiltrate" has at least ruled out common infectious agents and unusual dermatoses. A supportive pathologic diagnosis interpreted in conjunction with the clinical impressions may be just as useful as a confirmatory diagnosis.

Technique

Selection of the Site

✓ Selection of the site requires careful examination of the entire animal for the most representative samples, identification of the primary and secondary lesions present, and the formation of a list of differential diagnoses before biopsy.

⊶ With the exception of a solitary nodule, we recommend taking multiple tissue samples. These should include primary lesions if present, contain a representative range of lesions, and above all, should be taken and handled carefully. A normal sample of haired skin should also be included.

✓ Depigmenting lesions should be biopsied in an area of active depigmentation (gray color) rather than the final stage (white or pink color).

✓ Alopecia should be biopsied in the center of the worst area as well as in junctional and normal areas.

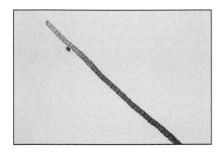

Figure 1-49
Hair tips are broken off in an alopecic cat with atopic dermatitis (original magnification x100).

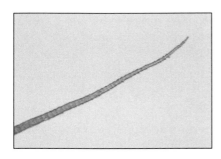

Figure 1-50
Tapered hair tips from an alopecic area of a dog with hyperadrenocorticism (original magnification x100).

✓ Ulcers and erosions should not be biopsied. Do not expect a pathologist to be able to describe more specifically than "an ulcer" if an ulcer is biopsied or "a crusted erosion" if an excoriated area is selected.

Preparation of the Site

✓ With the exception of excision biopsies of nodules, no surgical preparation of the site should be employed. Even topical application of alcohol and air drying may alter the epidermis.

🖐 If crusts are present, these should be left on the skin. If they are accidentally dislodged they should still be placed in the formalin and a note "please cut in crusts" should be added to the request form. Crusts may contain microorganisms or acantholytic cells that will help to obtain a diagnosis. Infection as a result of lack of surgical preparation does not seem to be a problem.

Wedge versus Punch Biopsy

✓ There are two commonly employed biopsy techniques in veterinary medicine—the punch biopsy and the wedge biopsy. The latter is commonly employed as an excisional technique when removing solitary nodules. It is also indicated with vesicles (which are typically too fragile to survive a punch biopsy with-

out rupturing), suspected cases of panniculitis (in which sufficient depth of biopsy may not be achieved with a punch) and
when biopsying the edge of a lesion in a spindle shape (which
allows correct orientation of the lesion in the laboratory where
spindle-shaped lesions are always cut in longitudinally).

✓ The punch biopsy is quick, relatively atraumatic, and usually
employed with suspected infectious, inflammatory, and endocrine dermatoses. Disposable biopsy punches are readily available in various
sizes. They can be cold-sterilized and reused.

✋ With the exception of face and foot biopsies, 8 mm punches
should be used! Smaller punches with a diameter of 4 or 6 mm are
employed to biopsy face and feet. Very small punches (i.e., 2 to 3 mm)
are not useful in small animal practice with the exception of eyelid
biopsies.

✓ The overlying hair is clipped and gently removed and the biopsy
site is marked with a water-proof marker pen (Figure 1-51). If crusts
are present, using scissors may be less traumatic.

✋ General anesthesia is indicated for nasal or footpad biopsies.
I use a combination of ketamine at 5 mg/kg bodyweight and diazepam
at 0.25 mg/kg body weight given intravenously in one syringe. No further preparation is necessary. If the biopsy is to be performed under
manual restraint or with sedation (I use xylazine at 0.4 mg/kg or
medetomidine at 10 mcg/kg intravenously), then a subcutaneous
injection of 1ml xylocaine (or the less stinging prilocaine) without
adrenaline will usually provide adequate local anesthesia (Figure 1-52).
If the agent is administered subcutaneously with the needle entry
point outside the proposed biopsy area, there should be no disruption
to the biopsy.

💣※ Don't overdose small animals with lignocaine (> 1ml / 5 kg), since
this can cause cardiac arrhythmias.

✋ Allow 3 to 5 minutes for the local anesthetic to have effect.

✓ If a punch is used, it is held at right angles to the surface of the skin
and gently placed over the selected lesion (Figure 1-53). Firm continu-
ous pressure is applied and the punch is rotated in one direction (note
carefully!) until a sufficient depth has been reached to free the dermis
from its underlying attachment. The punch is removed and any blood
should be carefully blotted.

✓ The section of tissue is grasped at the base—which should be the
panniculus—and subcutaneous attachments severed (Figure 1-54).
Under no circumstances should the dermis or epidermis be grasped
with forceps because this leads to a "crush artifact." Crushed tissue
may be misinterpreted as scarring at best, and at worst renders the
sample worthless. The tissue is rolled on gauze to gently blot the blood

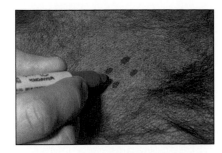

Figure 1-51
The biopsy site is gently clipped and marked with a water-proof marker pen.

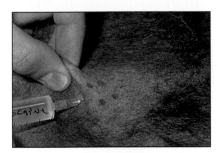

Figure 1-52
Local anaesthetic is injected subcutaneously.

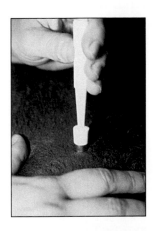

Figure 1-53
The punch is placed vertically onto the surface and rotated in only one direction.

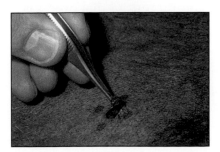

Figure 1-54
The sample is removed by grasping its base with a forceps and cutting it.

from its surface. A thin sample should then be placed with the panniculus face down—onto a rigid piece of cardboard or broken tongue depressor (Figure 1-55). This prevents the tissue from curling when placed in the formalin optimizing the interpretation by the pathologist. Thick samples may be placed in formalin without such support.

✓ The unit of tissue and cardboard is placed in 10% formalin (tissue side down) and allowed to fix for several hours before sectioning. The volume of formalin required is at least 10 times the volume of the sample. Nodules should be sectioned into 1 cm thick pieces to allow adequate penetration of the formalin into the center of the lesion.

Submission of Biopsy Samples

🖐 Careful completion of the appropriate skin biopsy request form, including history and physical examination, will greatly improve the chances of a diagnostic report.

🖐 A list of differential diagnoses is important with any clinical case but is essential with dermatologic patients. Seborrhea or draining tracts can be the result of a wide range of disease processes. This list is important for the clinician to ensure that he or she has considered all options and obtained as much information as possible from both pet and owner as necessary before taking the biopsy. It is also important for the pathologist and may aid in choosing special stains to rule out or confirm unusual diseases.

Serum Testing for Allergen-specific IgE

Indication

Useful if the owner of an atopic dog or cat diagnosed by history, clinical examination, and ruling out of differential diagnoses, is either curious about what causes the problem or is interested in allergen-specific immunotherapy.

Interpretation

✓ Different serum tests are available. Laboratory techniques have improved over the years and serum testing has become an alternative to intradermal skin testing for many small animal practitioners. However, tests vary in their sensitivity and specificity so that careful selection of an appropriate test is important.

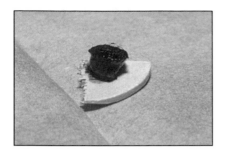

Figure 1-55
If the biopsy specimen is thin, it is placed
onto a cardboard or tongue depressor
before placing it into formalin.

✓ Testing for individual allergens rather than allergen groups is
prudent to avoid immunotherapy with inappropriate allergens. It
is impossible to tell which of the allergens in a particular react-
ing group are involved in the disease process.

✓ Results need to be interpreted in light of the clinical history of a
patient. A dog with positive reactions to grass pollens only and a clinical history of nonseasonal pruritus for years in a temperate environment such as in England or Canada will most likely not benefit from
allergen-specific immunotherapy.

✓ I still consider intradermal skin testing my first choice for the
identification of offending allergens in atopic dermatitis for several
reasons: 1) more individual allergens are used in skin testing than in
serum testing; 2) the skin is the affected organ and thus it seems
logical to test the organ affected; and 3) the input of a veterinary
dermatologist in regards to the interpretation of test results and management of patients on allergen-specific immunotherapy is invalu-
able for practitioners with limited experience in this particular field.

Bacterial Culture

Bacterial cultures are used infrequently in veterinary dermatology. Most
bacterial skin infections are caused by *Staphylococcus intermedius*. If cocci
are identified on cytology, empiric antibiotic therapy is sufficient in
almost all patients.

Indication

✓ Empiric therapy at appropriate doses for an appropriate time has
failed to resolve the pyoderma (lesions are still present and cytology
still reveals cocci).

✓ Numerous rod-shaped bacteria are identified on cytology samples from ear canals. These organisms may also rarely play a role in cutaneous infections of patients clinically not responding to empiric therapy.

Procedure

✓ Swabs are taken from ear canals as described for cytology samples.

✓ Aspirates from intact pustules are useful in patients with superficial pyoderma.

☞ Swabs from the skin surface to culture organisms from patients with deep pyoderma are not suitable. Samples are taken in a similar manner to that used in biopsies under aseptic conditions (scrub the skin surface and use sterile instruments and gloves). The upper half of the tissue sample with the epidermis and hair is cut off and the lower half is submitted in a sterile container placed on a sterile gauze pad soaked in a sterile saline solution for maceration culture. This prevents overgrowth of the culture by surface bacteria not relevant to the deep infection.

🖐 Each sample for culture and sensitivity should be accompanied by cytologic examination, and culture results must be interpreted in relationship to cytologic findings.

Patch Testing

This is the test of choice to confirm contact allergy. In classic patch testing, the test substance is applied onto intact skin (clipping is recommended 24 hours earlier, to minimize any confusion due to clipper rash in a sensitive individual), covered with an impermeable substance, and fixed. Human test kits are available (Figure 1-56). Alternatively, an area may be clipped and tape applied in a checkerboard pattern to leave two, four, or six spaces of bare skin surrounded by areas covered by tape (Figure 1-57). Then individual antigens are placed on to the bare patches and fixed with a tape. Fresh material may need to be cut up in small pieces and applied to the skin with the help of an ophthalmic lubricant gel. On top of this taped area, a whole trunk bandage is applied (and fixed around the neck as well) to avoid movement of the bandage and the allergens (Figure 1-58). After 2 days, the patch is removed and reactions are observed. After removing the bandage and allergens, the individual areas are marked with a permanent marker pen (to make possible a second evaluation 24 hours later). No reaction is graded as 0; erythema as 1+; erythema and edema or induration as 2+; and erythema and vesiculation as 3+.

The latter two reactions are considered significant. The bandage should then be reapplied (without taping and allergens) to avoid self-trauma and removed 24 hours later for a second evaluation. True contact allergy is characterized by a delayed-type reaction persisting or increasing during these 24 hours without the allergen on the skin.

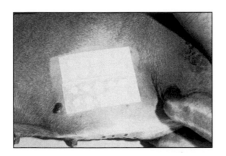

Figure 1-56
Human test kit on a dog. (Courtesy of Dr. Thierry Olivry.)

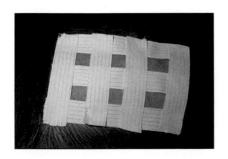

Figure 1-57
Patch test using tape.

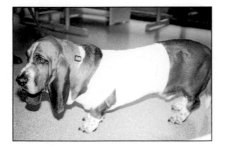

Figure 1-58
Trunkal bandage covering the patch test site.

If neither erythema nor vesiculation is present, the reaction on the previous day was probably caused by an irritant rather than allergic dermatitis. Topical or systemic steroids must be withdrawn for 3 to 6 weeks before testing.

In open-patch testing, the allergen is rubbed into a marked test site of normal skin and then examined daily over a 5-day period. The reactions similarly consist of mild erythema and edema. The technique is suitable only for liquid or plant allergens (in which crushed leaves are used). An already sparsely haired clinically unaffected area, such as the medial thigh or the inner pinna, is commonly used.

Diagnostic Trials

Diagnostic trials are well accepted tests in veterinary dermatology. They are performed when a certain problem is suspected and the trial is either the only or the best way to diagnose the possible underlying disease. A response to the trial confirms the diagnosis in some instances (such as the scabies treatment trial), but in other instances a relapse after discontinuing the trial with subsequent resolution on restarting the trial is diagnostic (such as in elimination diets). If there is no response to a well-conducted diagnostic trial, the suspected disease is extremely unlikely (which helps veterinarian, owner, and patient, and needs to be emphasized to clients frustrated by the lack of response).

Elimination Diet

Indication

An elimination diet is used to evaluate food adverse reaction which can occur with any food fed over a period of time. As a general rule food adverse reactions present infrequently. Any dog with nonseasonal pruritus (particularly if the face, feet, or ears are affected) or recurrent pyoderma, or any cat with miliary dermatitis, noninflammatory alopecia, eosinophilic granuloma complex, or head and neck pruritus could possibly have an underlying food adverse reaction.

Procedure

☞ An elimination diet for dogs consists of one protein source and one carbohydrate source previously not fed! This means that the elimination diet for a particular patient is determined by the diet fed so far to this animal. Cats are fed only one protein without the carbohydrate source to enhance compliance.

✓ Possible options for proteins are chicken, turkey, duck, venison, mutton, beef, horse, buffalo, rabbit, hare, kangaroo, emu, various sorts of fish, among others. Carbohydrates may consist of rice, potatoes, sweet potatoes, beans, or others.

✓ The diet chosen needs to be fed exclusively! Concurrent heart-worm prophylaxis or supplements must not contain food flavor extracts.

✓ It may take 6 to 8 weeks before a response becomes evident.

☞ After initial improvement, a rechallenge with the normal diet previously fed is essential because improvement may result from other factors such as seasonal or environmental changes or concurrent medication. If a relapse occurs within 2 weeks and clinical signs resolve again after reinstitution of the elimination diet, the diagnosis is confirmed.

Tips to increase compliance

✓ Warming the food may improve patient compliance.

✓ Spices such as garlic or salt (in small amounts) may also be beneficial to improve palatibility.

✋ If the animal (and owner) is used to treats, the habit should be continued in a modified fashion to prevent feeding of inappropriate proteins. Little pieces of the selected meat protein can be fried and kept in the fridge for use as treats. The selected meat can be dried (in the oven or microwave) and given as treats. If an animal is receiving potatoes in the diet, then fried pieces of potato may be used (so long as they are not fried in butter, but in a plant-derived oil). If rice is chosen, rice cakes may be an additional option.

✓ If bones are part of the normal diet, bones of the meat selected for the elimination diet may be fed if available.

✓ Good client communication is essential. It must be made clear that an occasional slip in feeding habits (as little as once or twice weekly of a very small amount of a different protein) may destroy all the effort.

✓ It may be worthwhile to advise neighbors about the diet as well.

✓ If a home-cooked diet is not an option, a commercial diet consisting exclusively of a protein source and a carbohydrate source not previously fed may be considered. The same principles apply to commercial as to home-cooked elimination diets. However, some animals with food adverse reactions may be missed when using commercial diets.

After a diagnosis of food adverse reaction is confirmed, the client has two options: 1. To continue a commercial elimination diet forever—the more convenient option; 2. A home-cooked diet. It should be properly balanced (the help of a veterinary nutritionist may be indicated).

✓ Identifying of the offending allergen allows a more varied diet and is achieved through a sequential rechallenge with proteins formerly fed. Beef, lamb, chicken, or cheese and milk products are added to the elimination diet one at a time for 2 weeks each. If a relapse occurs within the first 2 weeks (many patients show symptoms within the first 2 days), the protein is discontinued until the patient's condition settles. That particular protein is avoided in the future. After 2 weeks of a given protein without clinical symptoms, a reaction to this protein is ruled out and it may be fed in the future. Some dogs will tolerate any home-cooked diet, but relapse on commercial diets may be caused by a reaction to additives or preservatives.

Insect Control Trial

Indication

An insect control trial may be used in any patient with suspected insect-bite hypersensitivities. Most animals with insect-bite hypersensitivities will be allergic to fleas. Clients generally accept these trials more readily when they are labeled "insect control trials" because many do not believe fleas cause the problem, whereas most will accept ants or mosquitoes as a possible cause. Any dog with pruritus, alopecia, and/or a papular or crusty rash in the tailbase or inguinal area, and any cat with miliary dermatitis, noninflammatory alopecia, or eosinophilic granuloma complex may benefit from an insect control trial. Mosquito bite hypersensitivity in the cat is characterized by papules and crusts on the nose, pinnae, and foot pads. A trial using insect repellents may be beneficial to these animals.

Procedure

✓ The patient should be treated regularly with an insecticide. In a diagnostic trial, I often increase the frequency of administration above the manufacturer's recommendations. Fipronil spray, imidacloprid, permethrin, and selamectin spot-ons are administered every 2 weeks. Pyrethroid sprays are administered daily depending on the product. Nitenpyram tablets are given either daily or every other day. Which products to use depends on the individual circumstances. More details are provided on page 138.

✓ At the start of the trial, treat the animal's environment with an insect-development inhibitor such as methoprene, fenoxycarb, or pyriproxifen. More details are provided on page 138.

✓ Contact animals (either living in the same household or those that visit on a regular basis) must be treated as well, although the frequency between adulticide applications may be increased to the manufacturers' recommendations.

✓ At the start of the trial, I often prescribe 5 to 7 days of prednisolone at 1 mg/kg bodyweight daily to hasten clinical response.

If there is good response to the trial, insect-bite hypersensitivity is present and insect control may be tapered to the minimum required.

🖐 Remember that the required minimum treatment typically varies seasonally, as does the insect load.

Scabies Treatment Trial

Indication

Any pruritic dog or cat could possibly be infested with *Sarcoptes scabiei* or *Notoedres cati*, respectively, particularly if the pruritus was of sudden onset or if pinnae, ventrum, and elbows are pruritic. With spot-ons used for flea control, I have seen patients with pruritus and lesions limited to ventrum and lower legs. Negative superficial skin scrapings do not rule out scabies (p. 26) so trial treatment is indicated in any patient with suspected scabies irrespective of negative skin scraping results. In as much as *Cheyletiella spp.* and *Otodectes cynotis* are sensitive to the same antiparasitic agents, a scabies treatment trial will be useful for these parasites as well.

Procedure

✓ Several treatments for scabies are available but many of them are not labeled for this use.

✓ Topical treatments include ivermectin, lime sulfur dips, amitraz, and other antiparasitic rinses. They are used weekly for 4 weeks. More details are given on page 133.

✓ Systemic therapy may be undertaken with selamectin, ivermectin or milbemycin. Treatment details are outlined on page 133.

✓ All animals in contact with the patient need to be treated as well!

✓ Initial deterioration during the first days of treatment may occur. Treat with glucocorticoids daily for 3 to 4 days at 1 mg/kg body weight.

✓ Remission should be achieved within 4 weeks although some patients may need extended treatment for up to 8 weeks.

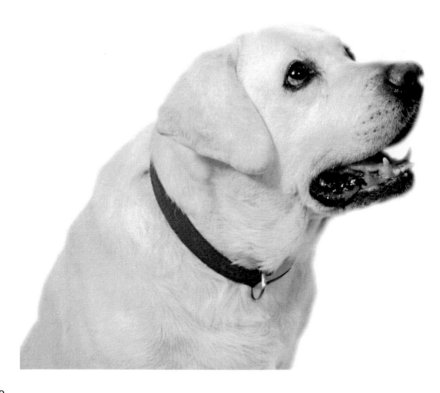

Section 2

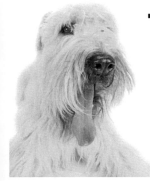

The Approach to Common Dermatologic Presentations

In this section, I offer an approach to various common presentations in veterinary dermatology. I begin each topic in this section with general comments followed by tables containing the most common differential diagnoses, their clinical features, diagnostic procedures of choice, treatment, and prognosis. I have attempted to list diseases in order of prevalence. Diseases marked with an (✱) and a colored screen are potentially difficult to diagnose or their management often requires considerable experience to achieve the best possible outcome. You may consider offering your client a referral to a veterinary dermatologist if you do not feel comfortable diagnosing or treating this disease.

This is not a textbook of veterinary dermatology so these tables do not contain all possible details but rather a concise overview concentrating on the most important features. Similarly, the flow charts at the end of each topic are concise and simplified to maximize the benefit for the busy small animal practitioner. They will be useful in most instances, but remember that some of your clients may not have read the textbooks. Even though this information is aimed at helping you as competent veterinarians to reach a diagnosis and formulate a treatment plan, your critical acumen, examination, and communication skills remain the most crucial instruments for success in your daily practice.

The Pruritic Dog

Key Questions

All questions discussed in Section 1 (pages 2-10) may be relevant for a pruritic patient.

Differential Diagnoses

If lesions are present, see page 58, The Dog with Papules, Pustules and Crusts. If no lesions are present, differential diagnoses are listed in Table 2-1.

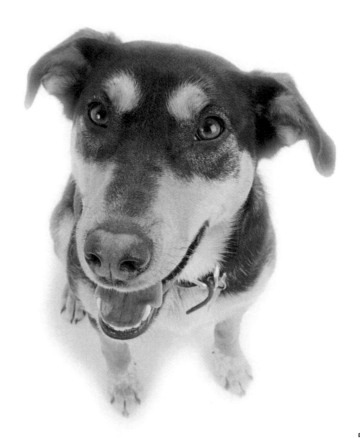

Table 2-1
Differential Diagnoses, Commonly Affected Sites, Recommended Diagnostic Tests, Treatment Options, and Prognosis in a Pruritic Dog Without Lesions

DISEASE	COMMONLY AFFECTED SITES	DIAGNOSTIC TESTS	TREATMENT	PROGNOSIS
Atopy* (Hypersensitivity to airborne allergens, such as pollens, house dust mites, or mold spores)	Face, feet, axillae, ears, ventrum, and perianal area (Figures 2-1, 2-2, and 2-3).	Diagnosis based on history, physical examination, and ruling out differential diagnoses! Intradermal skin test or serum test for allergen-specific IgE (p. 42) identify offending allergens and allow formulation of immunotherapy	Allergen-specific immunotherapy (p. 123), antihistamines (p. 125), essential fatty acids (p. 128), glucocorticoids (p. 129); shampoos (p. 115)	Good for well-being of the patient with continued, sometimes intensive management; guarded outlook for cure
Scabies (a highly contagious disease caused by *Sarcoptes scabiei var. canis*)	Pinnae, elbows, ventrum, hocks (Figures. 2-4 and 2-5).	Superficial skin scrapings (p. 26), Sarcoptes treatment trial (p. 49).	Antiparasitic agents such as amitraz, lime sulfur, ivermectin, or milbemycin oxime (p. 133)	Excellent
Malassezia dermatitis (an infection with *Malassezia pachydermatis* secondary to other skin disorders, such as allergies or endocrine problems)	Face, feet, ears, ventral neck, ventrum, and perianal area (Figures 2-6 and 2-7	Cytology (p. 21)	Antifungal agents such as ketoconazole (p. 131)	Good, but relapse likely if primary disease not addressed
Food adverse reaction (may or may not be allergic, commonly a reaction against a protein, rarely an additive, clinically indistinguishable from atopy)	Face, feet, axillae, ears, ventrum, perianal area (Figure 2-8)	Elimination diet (p. 46)	Avoidance, antihistamines (p. 125), essential fatty acids (p. 128), glucocorticoids (p. 129), shampoos (p. 115)	Excellent, if offending protein(s) is (are) identified and avoided, otherwise fair with continued management. Poor chance of cure

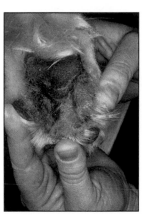

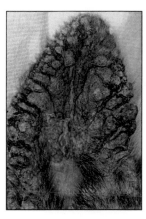

Figure 2-3
Pododermatitis in a
1-year-old, castrated
Golden Retriever with
atopy.

Figure 2-4
Severe pinnal crusting
in a 10-month-old,
female Akita with
scabies.

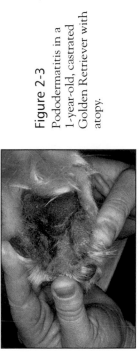

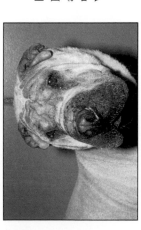

Figure 2-1
Facial erythema and
alopecia in a 5-year-old
male castrated Shar-pei
with atopic dermatitis.

Figure 2-2
Perianal alopecia,
erythema, and salivary
staining in an atopic,
2-year-old, female toy
Poodle.

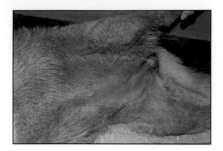

Figure 2-5
Ventral erythema, alopecia, and papules in the dog seen in Figure 2-4.

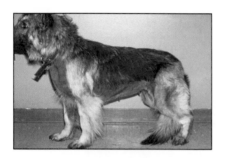

Figure 2-6
Hyperpigmentation and alopecia in a 2-year-old, spayed German Shepherd with *Malassezia canis*. (Courtesy of Dr. Thiery Olivry.)

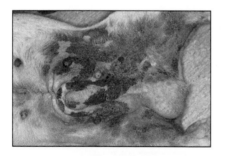

Figure 2-7
Malassezia-related dermatitis in a 9-year-old, male British Bulldog (Courtesy of Dr. Michael Shipstone.)

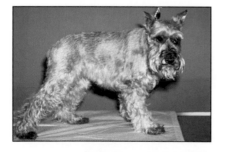

Figure 2-8
Pedal salivary staining in an 8-year-old, spayed Schnauzer with food-adverse reaction. (Courtesy of Dr. Peter Ihrke.)

Figure 2-9
The Nonlesional Pruritic Dog

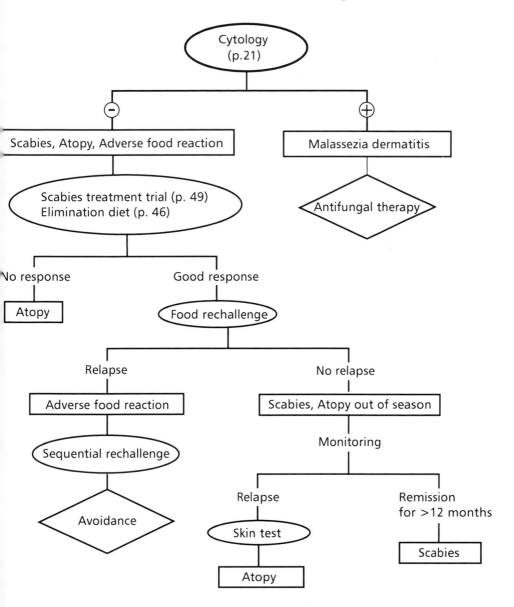

The Dog with Papules, Pustules, and Crusts

Key Questions

✓ What is the breed of this patient? (p. 2)

✓ How old was this patient when clinical signs were first recognized? (p. 3)

✓ How long has the disease been present and how did it progress? (p. 3)

✓ On which part of the body did the problem start? (p. 4)

✓ Is the animal itchy? (p. 5)

✓ Is the disease seasonal? (p. 6)

✓ Are there other clinical signs, such as sneezing, coughing, or diarrhea? (p. 7)

✓ What do you feed the animal? Was a special diet used in the past? (p. 7)

✓ Are there any other animals in the household? (p. 8)

✓ Does anybody in the household have skin disease? (p. 8)

✓ Was the disease treated before? If so, which drugs were used and how successful was treatment? (p. 8)

✓ What is used for flea control currently? (p. 9)

✓ When was the last medication given? (p. 9)

Differential Diagnoses

Papules may develop into pustules and crusts, and any dog with an acute papular rash may eventually show pustules or crusts. Some diseases are characterized by papules that do not typically develop further into pustules (such as flea-bite hypersensitivity); other diseases typically show crusting as their predominant symptom (such as zinc-responsive dermatitis). Tables 2-2, 2-3, and 2-4 list the major differential diagnoses for dogs with papules, pustules, and crusts. Lesions may be follicular or nonfollicular (Figure 2-10). Follicular papules and pustules indicate a pathologic process concentrating on the hair follicle, most commonly bacterial folliculitis, demodicosis, or dermatophytosis. Nonfollicular lesions may indicate pathologic processes concentrating on the epidermis, dermis, or dermo-epidermal junction, such as superficial spreading pyoderma, flea-bite, contact hypersensitivity, or immune-mediated skin diseases. Be aware that some nonfollicular processes may occasionally involve hair follicles as well.

Nonfollicular papule and pustule

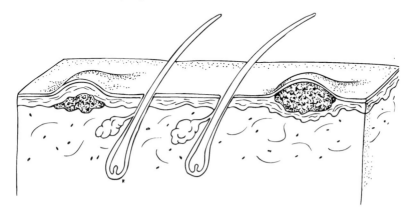

Follicular papule and pustule

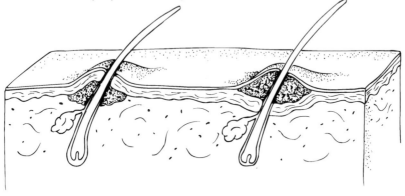

Figure 2-10

Table 2-2
Differential Diagnoses, Commonly Affected Sites, Recommended Diagnostic Tests, Treatment Options, and Prognosis in a Dog with Papules

DISEASE	COMMONLY AFFECTED SITES	DIAGNOSTIC TESTS	TREATMENT	PROGNOSIS
Flea-bite hypersensitivity (antigens in flea saliva injected during the flea-bite cause an allergic reaction in sensitized dogs)	Dorsal lumbosacral area, caudomedial thighs, inguinal area, ventrum, and perium-bilical area (Figures 2-11 and 2-12)	Flea control trial (p. 48) is best, serum or skin testing for allergen-specific IgE (only diagnostic in presence of type I hypersensitivity, dogs with delayed hypersensitivity to flea antigens provide negative results to serum tests, p. 42.)	Flea control (p. 136), antipruritic therapy (p. 123)	Fair to excellent depending on climate and owner commitment
Bacterial infection (typically by *Staphylococcus intermedius* and typically secondary to an underlying disease)	Erythema, scaling, seborrhea, alopecia, papules, pustules, and crusts, either focal or generalized depending on underlying disease (Figures 2-13 and 2-14)	Cytology (p. 21), biopsy (p. 38)	Antibacterial treatment (p. 118), shampoo therapy (p. 115)	Good, if underlying disease can be identified and treated appropriately. Relapse likely, if this is not possible
Demodicosis (probably a hereditary specific T-cell defect that permits abnormal proliferation of *Demodex canis*, a normal commensal mite of canine skin. This proliferation leads to a further parasite-induced immunosuppression. Adult-onset demodicosis frequently secondary to hormonal diseases, neoplasia, steroids, or other chemotherapy.)	Localized form: Focal erythema, alopecia and scaling, most commonly on the face (< 4 sites). Generalized form: Erythema, alopecia, papules, plaques, pustules and crusts where large areas, more than 5 areas, or paws are involved (Figures 2-15, 2-16, and 2-17)	Deep skin scrapings (p. 28), hair plucks (p. 36), biopsy (p. 38)	Localized form: 95% resolve spontaneously, thus benign neglect or antimicrobial treatment only (p. 119). Generalized form: Amitraz, ivermectin, milbemycin (p. 133), antibacterial treatment for secondary infection (p. 118)	Fair

Scabies (a highly contagious disease caused by Sarcoptes scabiei var. canis)	Pinnae, elbows, ventrum, and hocks	Superficial skin scrapings (p. 26), Sarcoptes treatment trial (p. 49)	Antiparasitic agents (p. 133)	Excellent
Dermatophytosis (dermatophytes are transmitted by contact with fungal elements)	Face, pinnae, paws (Figure 2-18)	Wood's lamp (p. 30), trichogram (p. 36), fungal culture (p. 32), biopsy (p. 38)	Antimycotic agents such as griseofulvin or ketoconazole (p. 131). Topical antifungal shampoos may decrease contamination of environment (p. 115).	Good
Contact hypersensitivity (delayed hypersensitivity reaction to environmental allergens, clinically overlapping with contact irritant dermatitis)	Erythema, macules, papules and/or vesicles in hairless or sparsely haired areas (scrotum, chin, perineum, palmar/plantar interdigital skin, ventral abdomen) (Figure 2-19)	Wood's lamp (p. 30), trichogram (p. 36), fungal culture (p. 32), biopsy (p. 44), patch testing (p. 44)	Avoidance, whole-body suits, pentoxyphylline at 15 mg/kg twice daily, glucocorticoids (p. 129).	Excellent with identification and avoidance of allergen, fair with medical management
Mast cell tumor*	Most commonly on the caudal half of the body (Figure 2-20)	Cytology (p. 21), biopsy (p. 38)	Surgical excision, sterile water injection, glucocorticoids (p. 129), chemotherapy, radiation.	Guarded

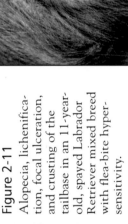

Figure 2-12
Alopecia and lichenification on the tail base of a 1-year-old, male Lhasa Apso cross with flea-bite hypersensitivity.

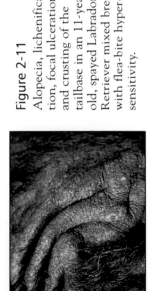

Figure 2-11
Alopecia, lichenification, focal ulceration, and crusting of the tailbase in an 11-year-old, spayed Labrador Retriever mixed breed with flea-bite hypersensitivity.

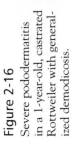

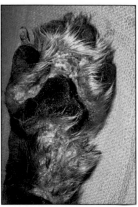

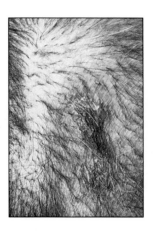

Figure 2-14
Crusted papules in a 3-year-old, male castrated Labrador Retriever with bacterial pyoderma.

Figure 2-16
Severe pododermatitis in a 1-year-old, castrated Rottweiler with generalized demodicosis.

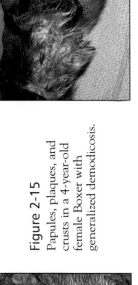

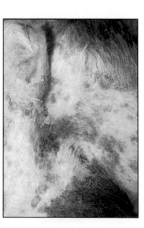

Figure 2-13
Papules, plaques, and epidermal collarettes in a 6-year-old, castrated Border Collie with pyoderma.

Figure 2-15
Papules, plaques, and crusts in a 4-year-old female Boxer with generalized demodicosis.

Figure 2-17
Abdominal papules in a 4-year-old, spayed Terrier mixed breed with generalized demodicosis.

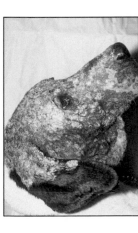

Figure 2-18
Severe crusting on the head of a 10-year-old, castrated Beagle mixed breed with dermatophytosis caused by *Trichophyton mentagrophytes*. Note the sharp demarcation between affected and nonaffected skin frequently seen with *Trichophyton* infections.

Figure 2-19
Papules and plaques resulting from contact hypersensitivity in a 3-year-old male Weimaraner. (Courtesy of Dr. Sonya Bettenay.)

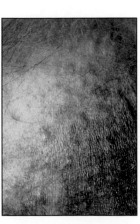

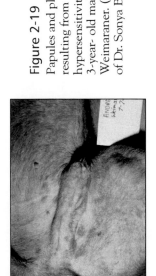

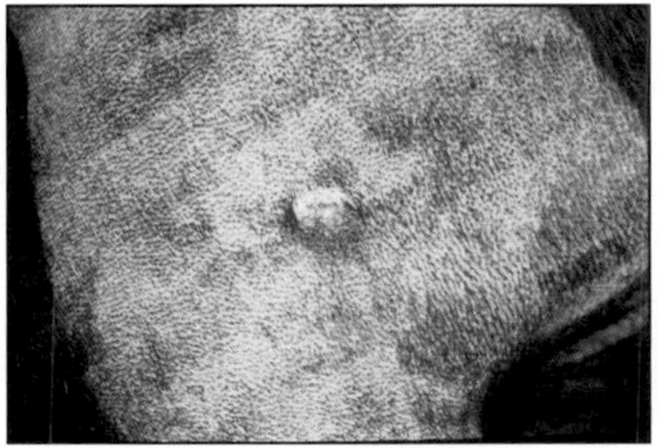

Figure 2-20
Mast-cell tumor in a 5-year-old, castrated Labrador Retriever.

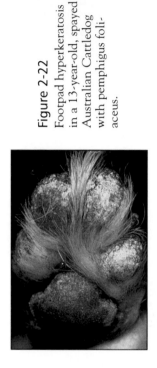

Figure 2-21
Papules, pustules, and crusting in a 6-year-old, castrated Labrador with severe pemphigus foliaceus.

Figure 2-22
Footpad hyperkeratosis in a 13-year-old, spayed Australian Cattledog with pemphigus foliaceus.

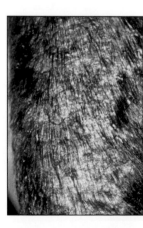

Table 2-3
Differential Diagnoses, Commonly Affected Sites, Recommended Diagnostic Tests, Treatment Options, and Prognosis in a Dog with Pustules

Disease	Commonly Affected Sites	Diagnostic Tests	Treatment	Prognosis
Flea-bite hypersensitivity (antigens in flea saliva injected during the flea-bite cause an allergic reaction in sensitized dogs)	Dorsal lumbosacral area, caudomedial thighs, inguinal area, ventrum, and periumbilical area (Figures 2-11 and 2-12)	Flea control trial (p. 48) is best, serum or skin testing for allergen-specific IgE (only diagnostic in presence of type I hypersensitivity, dogs with delayed hypersensitivity to flea antigens provide negative results to serum tests (p. 123)	Flea control (p. 136), antipruritic therapy (p. 123)	Fair to excellent depending on climate and owner commitment
Bacterial infection (typically by *Staphylococcus intermedius* and typically secondary to an underlying disease)	Erythema, scaling, seborrhea, alopecia, papules, pustules, and crusts, either focal or generalized depending on underlying disease (Figures 2-13, 2-14, and 2-15)	Cytology (p. 21), biopsy (p. 38)	Antibacterial treatment (p. 118), shampoo therapy (p. 115)	Good, if underlying disease can be identified and treated appropriately. Relapse likely, if this is not possible
Demodicosis (probably a hereditary specific T-cell defect that permits abnormal proliferation of *Demodex canis*, a normal commensal mite of canine	Localized form: Focal erythema, alopecia and scaling, most commonly on the face (< 4 sites). Generalized form: Erythema, alopecia, papules,	Deep skin scrapings (p. 28), hair plucks (p. 36), biopsy (p. 38)	Localized form: 95% resolve spontaneously, thus benign neglect or antimicrobial treatment only, p. 131).	Fair

64

induced immunosuppression. Adult-onset demodicosis frequently secondary to hormonal diseases, neoplasia, steroids, or other chemotherapy.)	where large areas, more than 5 areas, or paws are involved (Figures 2-15, 2-16, and 2-17)		ivermectin, milbemycin (p. 133), antibacterial treatment for secondary infection (p. 118)	Fair with appropriate treatment, poor for cure (except drug-triggered pemphigus)
Pemphigus foliaceus* (immune-mediated skin disease characterized by intraepidermal pustule formation due to pemphigus antibodies against antigens in the intercellular connections. May be idiopathic drug-induced or paraneoplastic)	Planum nasale, periocular area, lips, dorsal muzzle, inner surface of pinnae, foot pads, claw folds, nipples (in cats) (Figure 2-21, 2-22, 2-23, 2-43)	Cytology (p. 21), biopsy (p. 38)	Immunosuppression (p. 141)	

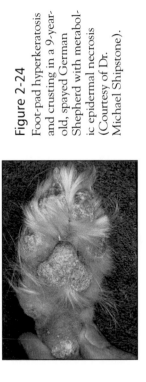

Figure 2-24
Foot-pad hyperkeratosis and crusting in a 9-year-old, spayed German Shepherd with metabolic epidermal necrosis (Courtesy of Dr. Michael Shipstone).

Figure 2-23
Large pustules in a 2-year-old, castrated Chow Chow with pemphigus foliaceus (Courtesy of Dr. Thierry Olivry).

Figure 2-25
Periocular erythema, alopecia, and crusting in a 4-year-old, female Husky with zinc-responsive dermatosis (Courtesy of Dr. Sonya Bettenay).

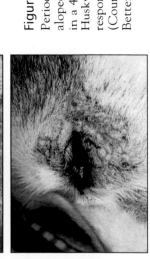

65

Table 2-4
Differential Diagnoses, Commonly Affected Sites, Recommended Diagnostic Tests, Treatment Options, and Prognosis in a Dog with Crusts

DISEASE	COMMONLY AFFECTED SITES	DIAGNOSTIC TESTS	TREATMENT	PROGNOSIS
Bacterial infection Flea-bite hypersensitivity (antigens in flea saliva injected during the flea bite cause an allergic reaction in sensitized dogs)	Dorsal lumbosacral area, caudomedial thighs, inguinal area, ventrum, periumbilical area (see Figures 2-11 and 2-12.)	Insect control trial (p. 48), serum or skin testing for allergen-specific IgE (only diagnostic in presence of type I hypersensitivity, dogs with delayed hypersensitivity to flea antigens are negative on serum tests, p. 42)	Flea control (p. 136), antipruritic therapy (p. 123)	Fair to excellent depending on climate and owner commitment
Demodicosis (probably a hereditary specific T-cell defect that permits abnormal proliferation of *Demodex canis*, a normal commensal mite of canine skin. This proliferation leads to a further parasite-induced immunosuppression. Adult-onset demodicosis frequently secondary to hormonal diseases, neoplasia, steroids, or other chemotherapy.)	Localized form: Focal erythema, alopecia and scaling, most commonly on the face (< 4 sites). Generalized form: Erythema, alopecia, papules, plaques, pustules and crusts where large areas, more than 5 areas, or paws are involved (Figures 2-15, 2-16, and 2-17)	Deep skin scrapings (p. 28), hair plucks (p. 36), biopsy (p. 38)	Localized form: 95% resolve spontaneously, thus benign neglect or antimicrobial treatment only, p. 131). Generalized form: Amitraz, ivermectin, milbemycin (p. 133), antibacterial treatment for secondary infection (p. 118)	Fair
Scabies (a highly contagious disease caused by *Sarcoptes scabiei var. canis*)	Pinnae, elbows, ventrum, and hocks	Superficial skin scrapings (p. 26), *Sarcoptes* treatment trial (p. 49)	Antiparasitic agents (p. 133)	Excellent
Pemphigus foliaceus* (immune-mediated skin disease characterized by intraepidermal pustule formation due to pemphigus antibodies against antigens in the intercellular connections. May be idiopathic drug-induced	Planum nasale, periocular area, lips, dorsal muzzle, inner surface of pinnae, foot pads, claw folds, nipples (in cats) (Figure 2-21, 2-22, 2-23, 2-43)	Cytology (p. 21), biopsy (p. 38)	Immunosuppression (p. 141)	Fair with appropriate treatment, poor for cure (except drug-triggered pemphigus)

66

Metabolic epidermal necrosis* (pathogenesis unclear)	Muzzle, mucocutaneous junctions, distal limbs, foot pads, elbows, hocks, ventrum (Figure 2-24)	Biopsy (p. 38)	Antimicrobial treatment, vitamin and mineral supplement, high-quality protein, intravenous amino acids	Poor
Dermatophytosis (dermatophytes are transmitted by contact with fungal elements)	Face, pinnae, paws (Figure 2-18)	Wood's lamp (p. 30), trichogram (p. 36), fungal culture (p. 32), biopsy (p. 38)	Antimycotic agents such as griseofulvin or ketoconazole (p. 131). Topical antifungal shampoos may decrease contamination of environment.	Good
Zinc-responsive dermatitis (Zinc deficiency due to insufficient zinc in the diet or insufficient absorption of zinc, especially in arctic breeds)	Periocular, perioral, pinnae, chin, foot pads, planum nasale, pressure points (Figure 2-25)	Biopsy (p. 38)	Zinc supplementation, low-dose glucocorticoids to increase zinc absorption	Fair
Idiopathic seborrhea* (primary keratinization defect as autosomal recessive trait with decreased epidermal cell renewal time and thus hyperproliferation of epidermis, sebaceous glands, and follicular infundibulum. Secondary to inflammation, endocrine disease, or nutritional deficiencies)	Otitis externa, digital hyperkeratosis, dry flaky skin, or seborrheic dermatitis predominantly on face, feet, ventral neck, and ventral abdomen (Figure 2-26)	Biopsy (p. 38)	Antiseborrheic shampoos (p. 115), moisturizers, retinoids, corticosteroids (p. 129)	Good to guarded for well-being, poor for cure.
Dermatomyositis (autosomal dominant in Collies and Shelties, first signs in puppies)	Erythema, scaling alopecia, mild crusting in face (particularly periocular area) eartips, carpal and tarsal regions, digits, tail tip, myositis, and in severe cases, megaesophagus	Skin biopsy, muscle biopsy, EMG	Vitamin E (200-800 iu/day), pentoxyphylline (20 mg/kg q 12 h), for acute flares prednisolone (1-2 mg/kg q 24 h)	Varies Dogs typically will not deteriorate further after 1 year of age.

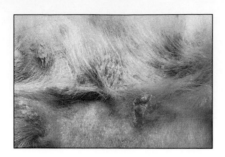

Figure 2-26

Crusted papules and plaques caused by idiopathic seborrhea in an 8-year-old, male castrated Cocker Spaniel.

Figure 2-27
The Dog with Papules, Pustules, or Crusts

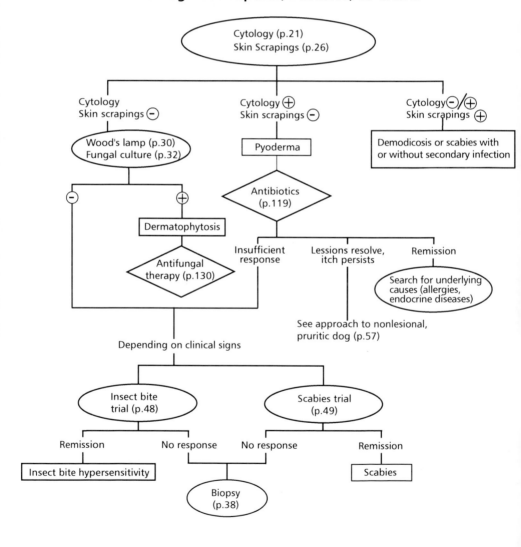

The Dog with Alopecia

Many diseases are associated with alopecia in conjunction with pruritus and other lesions. Here we discuss dogs with clinically noninflammatory alopecias.

Key Questions

✓ What breed is the patient? (p. 2)

✓ How old was this patient when clinical signs were first recognized? (p. 3)

✓ How long has the disease been present and how did it progress? (p. 3)

✓ On which part of the body did the problem start? (p. 4)

✓ Is the animal itchy? (p. 5)

✓ Is the disease seasonal? (p. 6)

✓ Are there other animals in the household? (p. 5)

✓ Does anybody in the household have skin disease? (p. 8)

✓ Was the disease treated before? If so, which drugs were used and how successful was treatment? (p. 8).

If the alopecic dog is pruritic but lacks other lesions, the approach is different from that used in a bald dog without pruritus. Many alopecias are characterized by dry skin and mild scaling, which may or may not be pruritic. The use of moisturizers will help the dryness and may address concurrent pruritus. If pruritus persists, then the approach is the same as for the dog with pruritus without lesions (p. 54). Differential diagnoses for noninflammatory and nonpruritic alopecias are outlined later in this section.

Table 2-5
Differential Diagnoses, Commonly Affected Sites, Recommended Diagnostic Tests,
Treatment Options, and Prognosis in Dogs with Noninflammatory, Nonpruritic Alopecia

DISEASE	COMMON SYMPTOMS	DIAGNOSTIC TESTS	TREATMENT	PROGNOSIS
Hyperadrenocorticism* (spontaneous or idiopathic) The spontaneous form is an excessive production of glucocorticoids due either to a microadenoma or macroadenoma of the pituitary gland – pituitary-dependent hyperadrenocorticism [=PDH], in 85% – or due to adrenocortical neoplasms in 15%)	Polyuria, polydipsia, polyphagia, dull haircoat, slow hair growth, coat color change, partial-to-complete symmetric alopecia of the rump, thin skin, recurrent skin and bladder infections, exercise intolerance, panting, muscle atrophy, anestrus, calcinosis cutis (Figure 2-28), behavioral changes, and neurologic signs (the latter with a pituitary macroadenoma)	Serum biochemistry (Serum alkaline phosphatase [SAP]↑, cholesterol ↑, alanine aminotransferase [ALT] ↑, glucose ↑, urea ↓), hemogram (leukocytosis, neutrophilia, lymphopenia, and eosinopenia), urinalysis (specific gravity ↓, cortisol:creatinine ratio ↑), radiographs (hepatomegaly, osteoporosis, mineralization of adrenal glands), low dose dexamethasone suppression test, adrenocorticotropic hormone (ACTH) in PDH ↑, ultrasonography (adrenal gland size ↑), ACTH stimulation test	Iatrogenic form: Cautiously taper and then discontinue glucocorticoid administration. Idiopathic form: o,p'-DDD (mitotane), ketoconazole for pituitary-dependent hyperadrenocorticism (p. 131), surgical removal of affected gland for adrenocortical neoplasia	Approximately 60% of dogs with adrenal tumors were reported to survive adrenalectomy and the postoperative period. The average life expectancy was 36 months. Adrenal adenomas have a better prognosis than adenocarcinomas. The life span of dogs with PDH treated medically averaged 30 months with some dogs living longer than 10 years and others only days.
Hypothyroidism (lymphocytic thyroiditis [presumably autoimmune] or idiopathic thyroid necrosis which may be end-stage lymphocytic thyroiditis)	Lethargy, obesity, depression, dull brittle coat, recurrent skin infections, thick, puffy skin (myxedema), hypotrichosis, alopecia (frictional areas, flanks, trunk, face), hypertrichosis (Boxers), seborrhea, neuromuscular symptoms, infertility	Serum biochemistry (SAP ↑, cholesterol ↑, ALT ↑), hemogram (anemia), thyroid tests (free thyroxine [T4], total T4, free T4 by equilibrium dialysis, thyroid stimulating hormone (TSH) assays, TSH stimulation test, thyrotropine-releasing hormone (TRH) stimulation test)	Hormone replacement therapy with levothyroxine (p. 144).	Good, although not all patients stay in complete and constant remission despite adequate supplementation

Follicular dysplasia (unknown etiology)	Noninflammatory alopecia sparing the head and limbs (Figure 2-29)	Biopsy (p. 38), ruling out endocrine disorders in equivocal cases.	Retinoids, melatonin (p. 144)	Excellent for well-being, guarded for hair regrowth
Cyclic follicular dysplasia (possibly related to duration of daily light exposure)	Seasonal local hyperpigmentation and alopecia of the trunk (often the flanks) with initially spontaneous regrowth after 3 to 4 months (Figure 2-30)	Biopsy (p. 38)	Melatonin (p. 144)	Excellent for general well-being, fair for prevention of hair loss with treatment
Pattern baldness (unknown etiology, probably genetically determined). Dachshunds and Greyhounds are predisposed	Alopecia of pinnae, postauricular region, ventral neck, ventrum, caudomedial thighs, tail (Figure 2-31)	Biopsy (p. 38), lack of endocrine abnormalities.	Benign neglect possibly in conjunction with moisturizers.	Excellent for well-being, poor for hair regrowth
Color dilution alopecia (genetically determined degenerative process resulting in lighter hair color with pigmentary clumping and damage to the hair shaft and bulb)	Alopecia of dilute blue or fawn colored areas, often with scaliness and recurrent folliculitis (Figure 2-32)	Cytology (p. 21), trichogram (p. 36), skin scrapings (p. 26), biopsy (p. 38).	Retinoids, essential fatty acid supplementation (p. 128).	Good for well-being, poor for hair regrowth
Growth hormone-responsive dermatosis, estrogen-responsive dermatosis, castration-responsive dermatosis, adrenal sex hormone imbalance, testosterone-responsive dermatosis, hypogonadism (unclear etiology in most of these syndromes that may be grouped together as "alopecia x")	Puppy-like hair coat, coat color changes, hypotrichosis and alopecia of the perineal and genital region, flank, trunk, neck (Figures 2-33 and 2-34)	Biopsy (p. 38) in conjunction with ruling out other endocrine disorders, such as hyperadrenocorticism and hypothyroidism, that may have similar histopathologic changes.	Benign neglect in conjunction with moisturizers and possibly antimicrobial treatment, neutering in intact dogs, testosterone in castrated males, estrogen in spayed females, growth hormone (diabetogenic), o,p'-DDD (risk of hypoadrenocorticism)	Good for well-being, treatment usually only leads to temporary remission

Table 2-5 continued

DISEASE	COMMONLY AFFECTED SITES	DIAGNOSTIC TESTS	TREATMENT	PROGNOSIS
Sertoli's cell tumor (most common in cryptorchid testicles, increased levels of estrogen)	Bilaterally symmetric alopecia of wear areas such as collar region, rump, perineum and genital area, gynecomastia, pendulous prepuce, linear preputial dermatosis, attraction of male dogs, prostatomegaly, prostatitis, estrogen-induced bone marrow suppression	Blood estrogen ↑, skin biopsy (p. 38), histopathologic evaluation of removed testes	Castration	Excellent with no metastases, guarded with metastases or aplastic anemia
Hyperestrogenism (Cystic ovaries or functional ovarian tumors)	Bilaterally symmetric alopecia of perineum, inguinal area and flanks, gynecomastia, and comedones, estrus cycle abnormalities	Biopsy (p. 38), blood estrogen ↑, ultrasonography, laparascopy	Ovariohysterectomy	Excellent
Anagen defluxion (severe systemic diseases or antimitotic drugs interfere with hair growth, resulting in abnormal hair shafts, hair breaks off suddenly)	Alopecia of sudden onset	History, trichogram (p. 36)	Addressing the underlying cause	Excellent if causative factor is addressed successfully
Telogen effluvium (severe stress [e.g. shock, fever, surgery] causes abrupt cessation of hair growth and switching to catagen and then telogen in many follicles, which are all shed simultaneously 1 to 3 months after the insult)	Focal to generalized alopecia of sudden onset	History, trichogram (p. 36).	Not needed, if stress was a one-time event	Excellent

Post-clipping Alopecia (arctic or plushcoated breeds fail to regrow hair in clipped areas; cause is unknown)	Clipped areas	Diagnosis based on signalment, history, and presence of noninflammatory alopecia in clipped areas only.	None. Hair will grow back in 6-24 months	Excellent

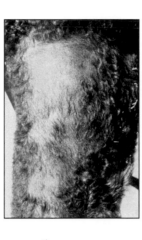

Figure 2-28
Papules and crusts in an 8-year-old, male castrated Bull Terrier with calcinosis cutis due to pituitary-dependent hyperadrenocorticism

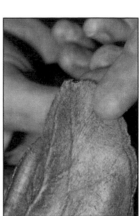

Figure 2-29
Alopecia due to follicular dysplasia in a 2-year-old, female Curly-coated Retriever

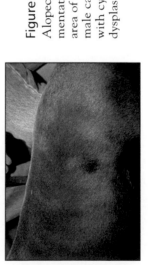

Figure 2-30
Alopecia and hyperpigmentation in the flank area of a 6-year-old, male castrated Boxer with cyclic follicular dysplasia.

Figure 2-31
Pattern alopecia. (Courtesy of Dr. Peter Ihrke.)

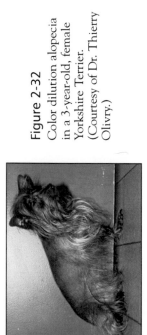

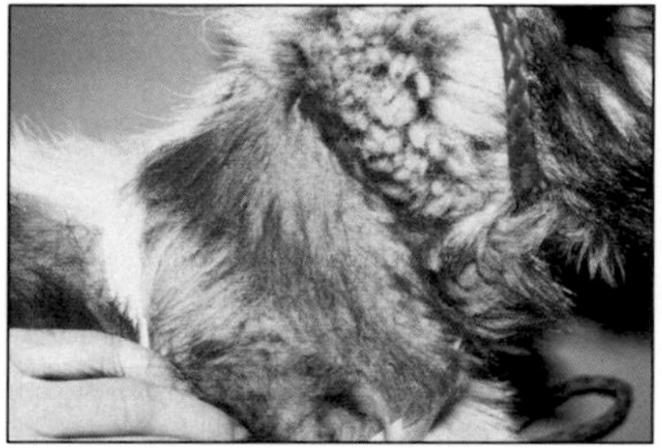

Figure 2-33
Growth hormone-responsive dermatosis in a 9-year-old, spayed Keeshond.

Figure 2-32
Color dilution alopecia in a 3-year-old, female Yorkshire Terrier. (Courtesy of Dr. Thierry Olivry.)

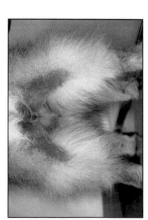

Figure 2-34
Castration-responsive dermatosis in a 5-year-old male Keeshond. (Courtesy of Dr. Sonya Bettenay.)

Figure 2-35

The Dog with Noninflammatory Nonpruritic Alopecia

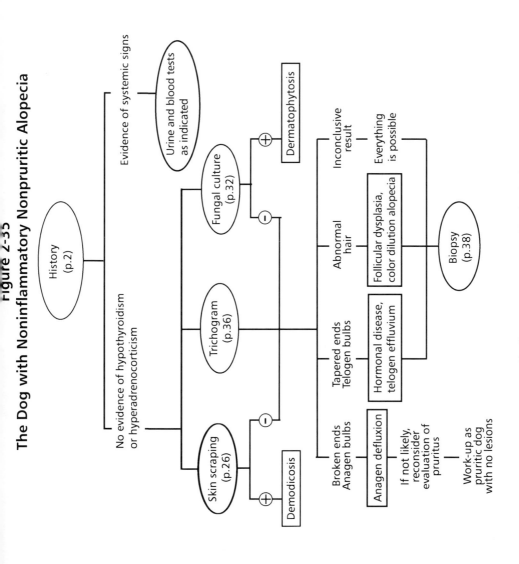

The Dog with Nodules

Key Questions

✓ How old was this patient when clinical signs were first recognized? (p. 3)

✓ How long has the disease been present and how did it progress? (p. 3)

✓ Are there any other animals in the household? (p. 8)

✓ Does anybody in the household have skin disease? (p. 8)

✓ Was the disease treated before? If so, which drugs were used and how successful was treatment? (p. 8)

Differential Diagnoses

The differential diagnoses are predicted primarily based on two separate features: (1) Is there only one lesion (which increases the likelyhood of neoplasia or a kerion) or are there multiple lesions (which may be due to sterile inflammatory diseases, more aggressive neoplastic disease or severe infection); and (2) Are draining tracts absent or present (increasing the likelihood of foreign bodies, severe bacterial or fungal infection, or sterile inflammatory disease)?

The approach to the dog with nodules is straightforward. History and clinical examination are followed by microscopical evaluation of impression smears (if draining tracts are present) and aspirates in any dog with nodules (p. 21). In some patients, cytology will reveal an infectious organism or classic neoplastic cells and thus a diagnosis. In most patients, cytologic examination will further narrow the list of differential diagnoses, but a biopsy (p. 38) will be necessary to reach a diagnosis. With nodular lesions, complete excision of one or more nodules should be performed. If draining tracts are present and/or cytology indicates possible infection, a culture may be useful as well. Deep tissue should be submitted rather than a culture swab (p. 28).

Table 2-6
Differential Diagnoses, Commonly Affected Sites, Recommended Diagnostic Tests, Treatment Options, and Prognosis in a Dog with Nodules

DISEASE	COMMONLY AFFECTED SITES	DIAGNOSTIC TESTS	TREATMENT	PROGNOSIS
Abscesses (caused by bite wounds or foreign bodies)	Fluctuating nodules most commonly around neck, shoulders and tailbase	Cytology (p. 21)	Surgical drainage, antibacterial treatment (p. 118)	Good
Neoplasia*	Varies with individual neoplastic diseases (Figures 2-36 and 2-37)	Cytology (p. 21), biopsy (p. 38)	Surgical excision and/or tumer specific therapy	Poor to excellent depending on the individual tumor
Sterile granulomatous and pyogranulomatous disease* (unknown pathogenesis)	Firm, painless, nonpruritic dermal papules, plaques and nodules typically of head, pinnae and distal limbs (Figure 2-38)	Cytology (p. 21), biopsy (p. 38), culture (p. 28, 32)	Doxycycline/Niacinamide (p. 121), immunosuppressive therapy (p. 141)	Fair with appropriate management
Sterile panniculitis* (mostly unknown pathogenesis, occasionally due to lupus erythematosus)	Solitary lesion over chest, neck or abdomen, multiple trunkal lesions with concurrent anorexia, lethargy, pyrexia (Figure 2-39)	Biopsy (p. 38)	Surgical excision for solitary lesions; vitamin E or systemic glucocorticoids for systemic disease	Fair with appropriate management
Opportunistic mycobacterial infection* (ubiquitous, facultatively pathogenic organisms, e.g., Mycobacteria fortuitum, M. chelonei, M. smegmatis cause lesions after traumatic implantation into subcutaneous tissue)	Nonhealing ulcerated nodules with draining tracts.	Biopsy (p. 38), culture (p.32)	Wide surgical excision followed by combination antimicrobial therapy (p. 131).	Fair to guarded

Table 2-6 continued

Disease	Commonly Affected Sites	Diagnostic Tests	Treatment	Prognosis
Dermatophyte kerion (caused by dermatophytes and secondary bacterial infection)	Nodular furunculosis with draining tracts (Figure 2-40).	Cytology (p. 21), biopsy (p. 38), fungal culture (p. 32).	Antimycotic and concurrent antibacterial therapy (p. 118)	Good
Cryptococcosis* (Rare infection in often immunocompromized host with ubiquitous, saprophytic, yeast-like fungus *Cryptococcus neoformans*)	Upper respiratory, cutaneous, central nervous and ocular signs. Papules, nodules, ulcers and draining tracts. Nose, lips, and claw beds maybe affected.	Cytology (p. 21), biopsy (p. 38), fungal culture (p. 32), serologic testing	Antimycotic therapy with amphotericin B possibly in combination with ketoconazole or itraconazole (p. 131)	Fair
Bacterial pseudomycetoma (nonbranching bacteria, such as coagulase-positive Staphylococci implanted during trauma, form grains of compact colonies surrounded by pyogranulomatous inflammation)	Firm nodules with draining fistulae	Cytology (p. 21), biopsy (p. 38), bacterial culture (p. 43)	Complete surgical excision, postsurgical antibacterial treatment (p. 118)	Fair with complete excision, guarded, if this is not possible
Sporotrichosis* (caused by ubiquitous dimorphic fungal saprophyte *Sporothrix schenkii* that infects wounds) Zoonosis, although zoonotic potential of canine sporotrichosis is much lower than that of feline sporotrichosis	Multiple nodules or ulcerated plaques on the head, pinnae, and trunk.	Biopsy (p. 38), fungal culture (p. 32)	Antimycotic therapy with iodides or azoles (p. 131)	Fair

Eumycotic mycetoma (ubiquitous soil saprophytes cause disease through wound contamination)	Nodules with draining tracts and scar tissue. Grains vary in size, shape, and color.	Cytology (p. 21), biopsy (p. 32), culture (p. 32)	Wide surgical excision followed by antimycotic therapy (p. 131) based on in vitro susceptibility testing.	Fair to guarded depending on surgical excision.
Phaeohyphomycosis* (wound contamination by ubiquitous saprophytic fungi with pigmented hyphae)	Often solitary subcutaneous nodules on extremities.	Cytology (p. 21), biopsy (p. 32), culture (p. 32)	Wide surgical excision followed by antimycotic therapy (p. 131) based on in vitro susceptibility testing	Guarded
Actinomycosis* (traumatic implantation of or wound contamination with filamentous, anaerobic Actinomyces spp., commensals of the oral cavity and bowel)	Subcutaneous swellings, possibly with draining tracts and yellow sulfur granules	Cytology (p. 21), biopsy (p. 32), culture (p. 32)	Surgical excision followed by long term antibacterial therapy (p. 118)	Guarded
Actinobacillosis* (oral commensal aerobic Actinobacillus ligneriesii is traumatically implanted, often through bite wounds)	Thick-walled abscesses of the head, mouth, and limbs that discharge thick pus with soft, yellow granules.	Cytology (p. 21), biopsy (p. 32), culture (p. 32)	Surgical excision or drainage and long-term antibacterial therapy (p. 118)	Guarded
Blastomycosis* (rare infection by the dimorphic saprophytic fungus Blastomyces dermatitides) Possible zoonosis (through wound contamination)	Papules, nodules, subcutaneous abscesses with draining tracts on face and feet. Concurrent anorexia, weight loss, coughing, dyspnea, ocular disease	Cytology (p. 21), biopsy (p. 38), fungal culture (p. 32)	Antimycotic therapy (p. 131)	Guarded to poor, if central nervous system (CNS) involved and poor for vision, if uveitis is present.
Coccidioidomycosis* (rare infection with dimorphic, saprophytic fungus Coccidioides immitis)	Papules, nodules, abscesses, and draining tracts over infected bones. Concurrent anorexia, weight loss, coughing, dyspnea, ocular disease, CNS signs possible	Biopsy (p. 38), fungal culture (p. 32).	Antimycotic therapy (p. 131)	Guarded (reported overall recovery rate 60%) to poor (with bone involvement)

Table 2-6 continued

DISEASE	COMMONLY AFFECTED SITES	DIAGNOSTIC TESTS	TREATMENT	PROGNOSIS
Histoplasmosis* (uncommon infection with dimorphic, saprophytic soil fungus *Histoplasma capsulatum*)	Papules, nodules, ulcers, and draining tracts. Concurrent anorexia, weight loss and fever, coughing, dyspnea, gastrointestinal and ocular disease	Cytology (p. 21), biopsy (p. 38), fungal culture (p. 32)	Antimycotic agents (p. 131)	Fair to good for dogs with pulmonary disease, guarded to grave for disseminated disease
Nocardiosis* (*Nocardia* spp. are soil saprophytes and cause respiratory, cutaneous, or disseminated infections)	Ulcerated nodules and abscesses, often with draining tracts, on the limbs and feet	Cytology (p. 21), biopsy (p. 38), culture (p. 32)	Surgical drainage and antibacterial therapy (p. 118) based on in vitro susceptibility testing	Guarded
Pythiosis* (infection with aquatic fungi by exposure of damaged skin to infected stagnant water)	Ulcerated nodules of the face and legs develop into boggy masses with ulceration and draining tracts	Biopsy (p. 38), culture (p. 32)	Wide surgical excision	Guarded to poor
Tuberculosis* (rare infection in small animals caused by *Mycobacterium tuberculosis*, *bovis* and rarely *avium*, predominantly respiratory and digestive lesions)	Ulcers, plaques, and nodules on head, neck, and limbs that discharge yellow-green pus with unpleasant smell	Radiographs, biopsy (p. 38), culture (p. 32)	Combination antimicrobial therapy (p. 131), frequent euthanasia due to public health concerns	Poor

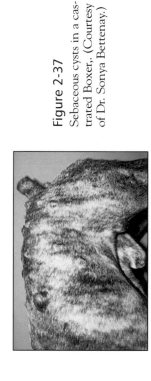

Figure 2-37
Sebaceous cysts in a castrated Boxer. (Courtesy of Dr. Sonya Bettenay.)

Figure 2-36
Histiocytoma in a 2-year-old castrated Jack Russell mixed breed.

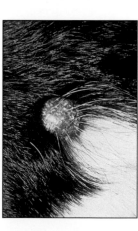

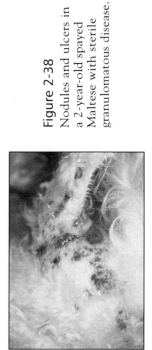

Figure 2-39
Sterile panniculitis with ulcers and nodules in a 9-year-old castrated English Springer Spaniel.

Figure 2-38
Nodules and ulcers in a 2-year-old spayed Maltese with sterile granulomatous disease.

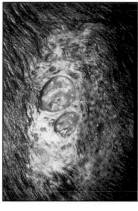

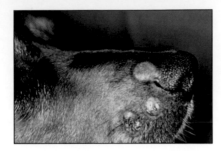

Figure 2-40
Dermatophyte kerion.
(Courtesy of Dr. Sonya Bettenay.)

Figure 2-41
The Dog with Nodules

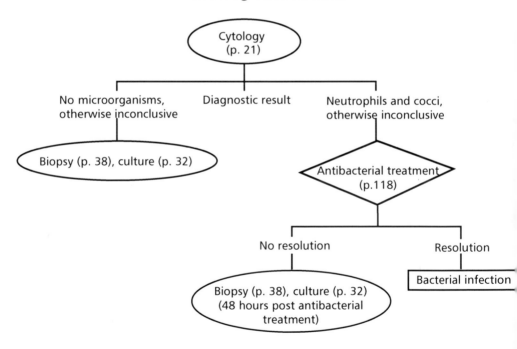

The Dog with Nasal Dermatitis

Key Questions

✓ How old was this patient when clinical signs were first recognized? (p. 3)

✓ How long has the disease been present and how did it progress? (p. 3)

✓ Is the disease seasonal? (p. 6)

✓ Are there any other animals in the household? (p. 8)

✓ Does anybody in the household have skin disease? (p. 8)

✓ Was the disease treated before? If so, which drugs were used and how successful was treatment? (p. 8)

✓ When was the last medication given? (p. 9)

Differential Diagnoses

Differential diagnoses are listed in Table 2-7. If lesions are present on the haired dorsal muzzle and the planum nasale, it is important to find out whether the first changes occurred on the planum nasale (possibly just as depigmentation) or in the haired skin. First changes in the haired skin indicate follicular diseases such as bacterial folliculitis, demodicosis, and dermatophytosis are more likely. If the planum nasale is affected first, immune-mediated skin diseases such as discoid lupus erythematosus or pemphigus foliaceus are higher on the list of possible conditions to be ruled out. If initial in-house tests such as skin scrapings (p. 26) and cytology (p. 21) are negative or nondiagnostic, biopsy (p. 38) is the next step.

Table 2-7
Differential Diagnoses, Commonly Affected Sites, Recommended Diagnostic Tests, Treatment Options, and Prognosis in a Dog with Nasal Dermatitis

DISEASE	AFFECTED SITES	DIAGNOSTIC TESTS	TREATMENT	PROGNOSIS
Discoid lupus erythematosus* (Immune-mediated reaction against basal cell layer may be aggravated by UV-light exposure)	Planum nasale, periocular area, lips, dorsal muzzle, pinnae (Figure 2-42)	Biopsy (p. 38)	Sun avoidance, water-proof sun screens, vitamin E (200-400 mg q 12 hr), doxycycline and niacinamide (p. 121), immunosuppressive therapy (p. 141)	Fair
Pemphigus foliaceus (Immune mediated reaction against dismonormal proteins)	Planum nasale, periocular area, lips, dorsal muzzle, inner surface of pinnae, foot pads, groin, claw folds, nipples (in cats) (Figures 2-21, 2-22, 2-23, and 2-43)	Biopsy (p. 38)	Immunosuppressive therapy (p. 141)	Fair
Bacterial infection (typically by *Staphylococcus intermedius* and typically secondary to an underlying disease)	Depigmentation of planum nasale in German Shepherd Dogs with atopy (Figure 2-44)	Cytology (p. 21), biopsy (p. 38)	Antibacterial treatment (p. 118)	Good, if underlying disease can be identified and treated appropriately. Relapse likely, if this is not possible
Demodicosis (probably a hereditary specific T-cell defect that permits abnormal proliferation of *Demodex canis*, a normal commensal mite of canine skin. This proliferation leads to a further parasite-induced immunosuppression. Adult-onset demodicosis frequently secondary to hormonal diseases, neoplasia, steroids, or other chemotherapy.)	Localized form: Focal erythema, alopecia and scaling, most commonly on the face (< 4 sites). Generalized form: Erythema, alopecia, papules, plaques, pustules and crusts where large areas, more than 5 areas, or paws are involved (Figures 2-15, 2-16, and 2-17)	Deep skin scrapings (p. 28), hair plucks (p. 36), biopsy (p. 38), elimination diet (p. 46)	Localized form: 95% resolve spontaneously, thus benign neglect or antimicrobial treatment only (p. 118). Generalized form: Amitraz, ivermectin, milbemycin (p. 133), antibacterial treatment for secondary infection (p. 118)	Fair

Dermatophytosis (dermatophytes are transmitted by contact with fungal elements)	Face, pinnae, paws (Figure 2-18)	Wood's lamp (p. 30), trichogram (p. 36), fungal culture (p. 32), biopsy (p. 38)	Antimycotic agents such as griseofulvin or ketoconazole (p. 131). Topical antifungal shampoos may decrease contamination of environment.	Good
Sporotrichosis* (caused by ubiquitous dimorphic fungal saprophyte *Sporothrix schenkii* that infect wounds) Zoonosis, although zoonotic potential of canine sporotrichosis is much lower than that of feline sporotrichosis	Multiple nodules or ulcerated plaques on the head, pinnae, and trunk.	Biopsy (p. 38), fungal culture (p. 32)	Antimycotic therapy with iodides or azoles (p. 131)	Fair
Cryptococcosis* (Rare infection in often immunocompromised host with ubiquitous, saprophytic, yeast-like fungus *Cryptococcus neoformans*)	Upper respiratory, cutaneous, central nervous and ocular signs. Papules, nodules, ulcers and draining tracts. Nose, lips, and claw beds maybe affected.	Cytology (p. 21), biopsy (p. 38) fungal culture (p. 32), serologic testing	Antimycotic therapy with amphotericin B possibly in combination with ketoconazole or itraconazole (p. 131)	Fair

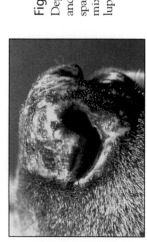

Figure 2-42

Depigmentation, erosions, and ulcers in a 3-year-old spayed Australian Shepherd mixed breed with discoid lupus erythematosus.

85

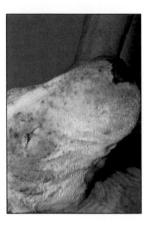

Figure 2-43
Pemphigus foliaceus with depigmentation, erosions, and crusting in a 7-year-old male Golden Retriever.

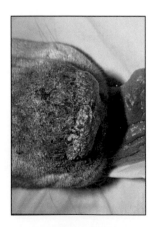

Figure 2-44
Bacterial facial and nasal pyoderma in a 5-year-old castrated Bull Terrier. Note that the planum nasale is spared. (Courtesy of Dr. Sonya Bettenay.)

**Figure 2-45
The Dog with Nasal Dermatitis**

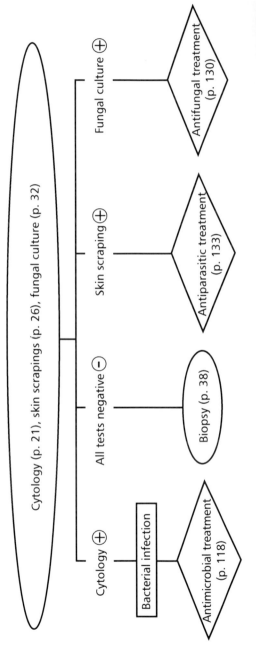

Cytology (p. 21), skin scrapings (p. 26), fungal culture (p. 32)

Cytology ⊕ — Bacterial infection → Antimicrobial treatment (p. 118)

All tests negative ⊖ → Biopsy (p. 38)

Skin scraping ⊕ → Antiparasitic treatment (p. 133)

Fungal culture ⊕ → Antifungal treatment (p. 130)

The Cat with Miliary Dermatitis

Key Questions

✓ How old was this patient when clinical signs were first recognized? (p. 3)

✓ How long has the disease been present and how did it progress? (p. 3)

✓ On which part of the body did the problem start? (p. 4)

✓ Is the disease seasonal? (p. 6)

✓ Are there other clinical signs such as sneezing, coughing, or diarrhea? (p. 7)

✓ What do you feed the animal? Was a special diet used in the past? (p. 7)

✓ Are there any other animals in the household? (p. 8)

✓ Does anybody in the household have skin disease? (p. 8)

✓ Was the disease treated before? If so, which drugs were used and how successful was treatment? (p. 8)

✓ What is used for flea control now? (p. 9)

✓ When was the last medication given? (p. 9)

Differential Diagnoses

Classic lesions of miliary dermatitis are focal or generalized small papules and crusts (Figures 2-46 and 2-47). Miliary dermatitis is not a diagnosis but rather a descriptive term for a feline cutaneous reaction pattern with many possible causes. Most cats suffer from an underlying flea-bite hypersensitivity. The differential diagnoses for feline miliary dermatitis are listed in Table 2-8.

Table 2-8
Differential Diagnoses, Commonly Affected Sites, Recommended Diagnostic Tests, Treatment Options, and Prognosis in a Cat with Miliary Dermatitis

Disease	Commonly Affected Sites	Diagnostic Tests	Treatment	Prognosis
Flea-bite hypersensitivity	Dorsal lumbosacral area, caudal half of the body or generalized disease (Figures 2-46 and 2-47)	Flea control trial (p. 48)	Flea control (p. 136), glucocorticoids (p. 129), antihistamines (p. 129), essential fatty acids (p. 128).	Good for well-being of the patient with continued management; guarded for cure
Atopy* (hypersensitivity to aeroallergens such as pollens, house dust mites or mold spores)	Head and neck, generalized disease.	Diagnosis based on history, physical examination and ruling out differential diagnoses. Intradermal skin test allows formulation of immunotherapy	Allergen-specific immunotherapy (p.123), antihistamines (p. 125), essential fatty acids (p. 128), glucocorticoids p. 129).	Good for well-being of the patient with continued management; guarded for cure
Food adverse reaction (may or may not be allergic, commonly reaction against a protein, rarely an additive, clinically indistinguishable from atopy)	Cranial half of the body or generalized disease	Elimination diet (p. 46)	Avoidance, antihistamines (p. 125), essential fatty acids (p. 128), glucocorticoids (p. 129).	Excellent, if offending protein(s) is (are) identified and avoided. Only fair with continued management, if not. Guarded for cure
Mosquito-bite hypersensitivity (an allergic reaction to salivary antigens of mosquitoes)	Papules and crusts on dorsal muzzle, lateral aspects of pinnae, and foot pads (Figures 2-48 and 2-49)	Keeping cat indoors for some days, biopsy (p. 38)	Indoor confinement (at least during dusk and dawn), insect repellents such as pyrethrine sprays.	Good for well-being of the patient with continued management; guarded for cure
Bacterial superficial folliculitis (caused by Staphylococci and secondary to other diseases)	Head and neck or generalized	Cytology (p. 21), biopsy (p. 38)	Antibacterial agents (p. 119)	Good, but relapse likely if underlying disease is not identified and treated

Otodectes cynotis infestation (may cause more than just otitis externa)	Otitis externa, pinnae, face, neck, thighs, tail, and tailbase	Superficial skin scrapings (p. 26), miticidal treatment trial (p. 49)	Antiparasitic agents (p. 133)	Excellent
Pemphigus foliaceus*	Yellowish to brownish crusts may be mistaken for the typically smaller and darker classical miliary dermatitis lesions. Head, inner pinnae, claw beds, nipples	Cytology (p. 21), biopsy (p. 38)	Immunosuppression (p. 141)	Fair
Mast cell tumor*	Papular form may occasionally be mistaken for miliary dermatitis	Cytology (p. 21), biopsy (p. 38)	Glucocorticoids (p. 129), chemotherapy	Fair
Dermatophytosis (in this form typically caused by M. canis)	Focal or generalized	Cytology (p. 21), Wood's lamp (p. 30), fungal culture (p. 32), biopsy (p. 38)	Antifungal agents (p. 130)	Guarded for cure in catteries and Persian cats, good otherwise.
Cheyletiellosis (Depending on location a rare to common contagious disease caused by Cheyletiella blakei)	Typically characterized by excessive scaling particularly on the dorsum, but occasionally generalized miliary dermatitis	Superficial skin scrapings (p. 26), sarcoptes treatment trial (p. 49), flea combing and microscopically evaluating debris covered with mineral oil in a Petri dish	Antiparasitic agents (p. 133)	Excellent
Feline scabies (a highly contagious disease caused by Notoedres cati)	Pinnae, face, neck, generalized disease.	Superficial skin scrapings (p. 26), sarcoptes treatment trial (p. 49)	Antiparasitic agents (p. 133)	Excellent

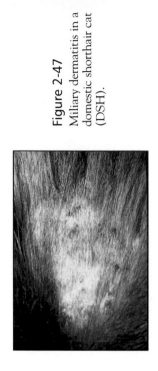

Figure 2-47
Miliary dermatitis in a domestic shorthair cat (DSH).

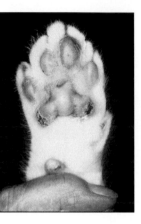

Figure 2-49
Crusting on the edges of the footpads due to mosquito-bite hypersensitivity in a 5-year-old spayed DSH. (Courtesy of Dr. Sonya Bettenay.)

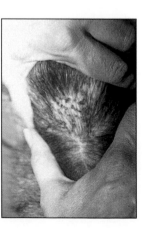

Figure 2-46
Erosions and crusted papules in a cat with miliary dermatitis.

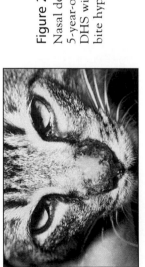

Figure 2-48
Nasal dermatitis in a 5-year-old castrated DHS with mosquito-bite hypersensitivity.

Figure 2-50
The Cat with Miliary Dermatitis

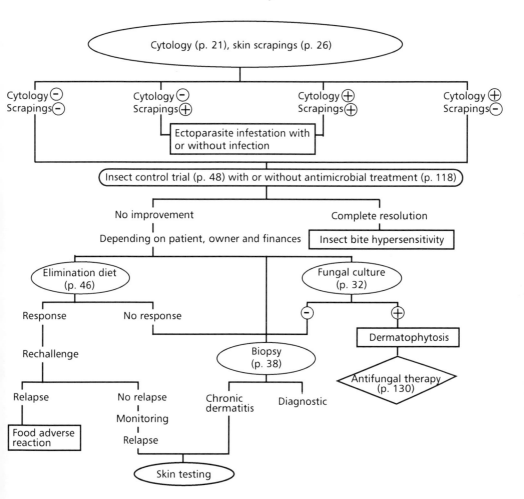

The Cat with Noninflammatory Alopecia

Key Questions:

✓ How old was this patient when clinical signs were first recognized? (p. 3)

✓ How long has the disease been present and how did it progress? (p. 3)

✓ On which part of the body did the problem start? (p. 4)

✓ Is the disease seasonal? (p. 6)

✓ Are there other clinical signs such as sneezing, coughing or diarrhea? (p. 7)

✓ What do you feed the animal? Was a special diet used in the past? (p. 7)

✓ Are there any other animals in the household? (p. 8)

✓ Does anybody in the household have skin disease? (p. 8)

✓ Was the disease treated before? If so, which drugs were used and how successful was treatment? (p. 8)

✓ What is used for flea control now? (p. 9)

✓ When was the last medication given? (p. 9)

Differential Diagnoses

Noninflammatory alopecia is a feline cutaneous reaction pattern that may have various causes. Hormonal alopecia is extremely rare in the feline and typically affected cats show other severe signs. Psychogenic alopecia in the cat is greatly overdiagnosed. The disease usually affects pure-bred cats with a nervous disposition. Environmental changes such as a new partner, baby, pet, or a move to a new house precede clinical signs. Most cats with noninflammatory alopecia are pruritic as a result of allergies and may be closet groomers. Many cats previously diagnosed with hormonal alopecia and treated successfully with medroxyprogesteron acetate or megestrol acetate have responded because the anti-inflammatory action of these medications have controlled their pruritus caused by allergies, not because of a correction of their hormonal imbalance. The differential diagnoses for feline noninflammatory alopecia are listed in Table 2-9.

Table 2-9
Differential Diagnoses, Commonly Affected Sites, Recommended Diagnostic Tests, Treatment Options, and Prognosis in a Cat with Noninflammatory Alopecia

DISEASE	COMMONLY AFFECTED SITES	DIAGNOSTIC TESTS	TREATMENT	PROGNOSIS
Flea-bite hypersensitivity	Dorsal lumbosacral area, caudal half of the body or generalized disease	Trichogram (p. 36), flea control trial (p. 48)	Flea control (p. 136), glucocorticoids (p. 129), antihistamines (p. 125), essential fatty acids (p. 128)	Good for well-being of the patient with continued management; guarded for cure.
Atopy* (hypersensitivity to aeroallergens such as pollens, house dust mites, or mold spores)	Cranial half of the body, ventrum, flanks or generalized disease (Figure 2-51)	Diagnosis based on history, physical examination, trichogram (p. 36) and ruling out differential diagnoses. Intradermal skin test allows formulation of immunotherapy	Allergen-specific immunotherapy (p. 123), antihistamines (p. 125), essential fatty acids (p. 128), glucocorticoids (p. 129)	Good for well-being of the patient with continued management; guarded for cure.
Food adverse reaction (may or may not be allergic, commonly reaction to a protein, rarely an additive, clinically indistinguishable from atopy)	Cranial half of the body, ventral abdomen or generalized disease	Trichogram (p. 36), elimination diet (p. 46)	Avoidance, antihistamines (p. 125), essential fatty acids (p. 128), glucocorticoids (p. 129)	Excellent, if offending protein(s) is (are) identified and avoided. Fair with continued management, if offending proteins are not identified. Guarded for cure.
Dermatophytosis (in this form typically caused by *M. canis*)	Focal or generalized	Trichogram (p. 36), cytology (p. 21), Wood's lamp (p. 30), fungal culture (p. 32), biopsy (p. 38)	Antifungal agents (p. 131)	Poor for catteries and Persians, good otherwise.
Psychogenic alopecia (due to excessive grooming caused by psychological factors)	Medial forelegs, caudal abdomen, inguinal region.	History (p. 2), trichogram (p. 36)	Environmental changes, glucocorticoids (p. 129), anxiolytic drugs.	Fair

93

Table 2-9 continued

DISEASE	COMMONLY AFFECTED SITES	DIAGNOSTIC TESTS	TREATMENT	PROGNOSIS
Hyperadrenocorticism* (very rare, similar pathogenesis to same condition in dogs)	Polydipsia, polyuria, weight loss, anorexia, polyphagia, depression, muscle wasting, alopecia (flanks, ventrum, or entire trunk), fragile skin	Ultrasonography, ACTH stimulation test, low-dose dexamethasone suppression test	Metyrapone, o,p -DDD, ketoconazole have been used	Poor
Anagen defluxion (severe diseases or antimitotic drugs interfere with hair growth, resulting in abnormal hair shafts, which causes hair to break off suddenly)	Alopecia of sudden onset	History, trichogram (p. 36)	Addressing the underlying cause	Excellent if causative factor is removed
Telogen effluvium (severe stress, such as shock, fever, surgery causes abrupt cessation of hair growth and switching to catagen and then telogen phases in many follicles, which are all shed simultaneously 1 to 3 months after the insult)	Focal to generalized alopecia	History, trichogram (p. 36)	Not needed, if stress was a singular event	Excellent

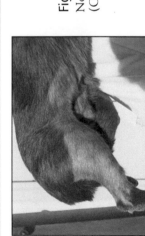

Figure 2-51
Noninflammatory alopecia in a cat with atopy.
(Courtesy of Dr. Wayne Rosenkrantz.)

Figure 2-52
The Cat with Noninflammatory Alopecia

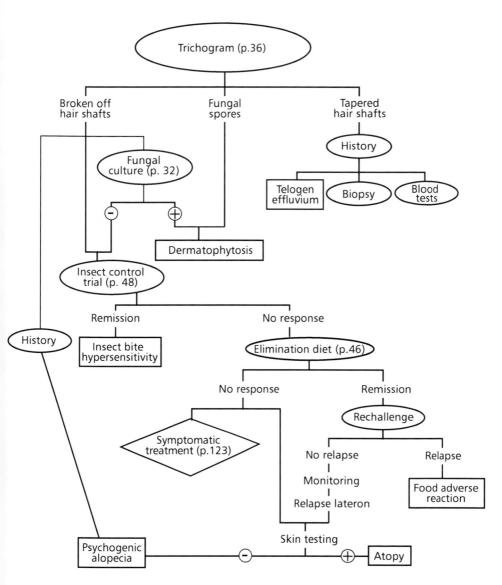

The Cat with Lesions of the Eosinophilic Granuloma Complex

Key Questions

✔ How old was this patient when clinical signs were first recognized? (p. 3)

✔ Is the disease seasonal? (p. 6)

✔ Are there other clinical signs such as sneezing, coughing, or diarrhea? (p. 7)

✔ What do you feed the animal? Was a special diet used in the past? (p. 7)

✔ Was the disease treated before? If so, which drugs were used and how successful was treatment? (p. 8)

✔ What is used for flea control now? (p. 9)

✔ When was the last medication given? (p. 9)

Differential Diagnoses

All subsets of the eosinophilic granuloma are mucocutaneous reaction patterns in the cat.

✔ Indolent (or eosinophilic or rodent) ulcer commonly affects the upper lip unilaterally or bilaterally (Figure 2-53), but may occur in the oral cavity or elsewhere on the body (Figure 2-54). The well-circumscribed ulcers with raised borders are rarely painful or pruritic; frequently the owner is more bothered by the lesions than the cat. The differential diagnoses of the feline eosinophilic ulcer are neoplastic diseases such as squamous cell carcinoma and infectious ulcers (eosinophilic ulcers are often secondarily infected as well). Diagnosis is confirmed by biopsy (p. 38). Prior antimicrobial treatment (p. 118) is recommended if cytology (p. 21) is indicative of infection.

✓ Eosinophilic plaques occur typically on the abdomen or medial thighs, are well-circumscribed, and severely pruritic (Figure 2-55).

✓ Eosinophilic (linear) granulomas are nonpruritic, raised, firm, yellowish, and clearly linear plaques and occur most commonly on the caudal thighs (Figure 2-56).

Differential diagnoses of both eosinophilic plaques and granulomas include neoplasias and bacterial and fungal granulomas (Table 2-10). Diagnostic procedures of choice are cytology (p. 21) and biopsy (p. 38). After the diagnosis has been confirmed, the underlying cause needs to be identified, if possible, and treated.

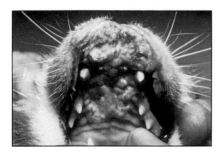

Figure 2-53
Indolent ulcer in a 2-year-old female DSH.

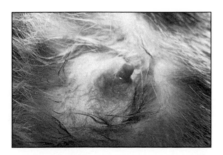

Figure 2-54
Indolent ulcer of the nipple in a 4-year-old female DSH.

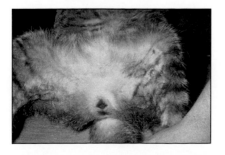

Figure 2-55
Eosinophilic plaques in the inguinal area of a DSH. (Courtesy of Dr. Sonya Bettenay.)

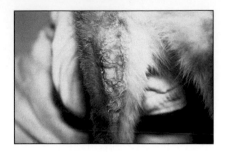

Figure 2-56
Linear granuloma in a male 8-year-old DSH.

Table 2-10
Underlying Causes and Recommended Diagnostic Tests in a Cat with Lesions of the Eosinophilic Granuloma Complex

DISEASE	DIAGNOSTIC TESTS	TREATMENT
Flea-bite hypersensitivity	Flea control trial (p. 136)	Flea control (p. 136), glucocorticoids (p. 129), antihistamines (p. 125), essential fatty acids (p. 128)
Atopy (hypersensitivity to aero-allergens such as pollens, house dust mites, or mold spores)	Diagnosis based on history, physical examination and ruling out differential diagnoses. Intradermal skin test allows formulation of immunotherapy.	Allergen-specific immunotherapy (p. 123), antihistamines (p. 125), essential fatty acids (p.128), glucocorticoids (p. 129)
Food adverse reaction (may or may not be allergic, commonly reaction to a protein, rarely an additive, clinically indistinguishable from atopy)	Elimination diet (p. 46)	Avoidance, antihistamines (p. 125), essential fatty acids (p. 128), glucocorticoids (p. 129)
Idiopathic eosinophilic granuloma (most likely genetic basis)	Ruling out possible hypersensitivities	Glucocorticoids (p. 129), antibiotics (p. 119)

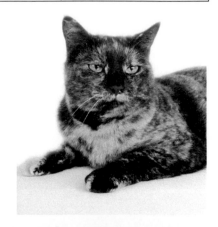

Figure 2-57
The Cat with Lesions of the Eosinophilic Granuloma Complex

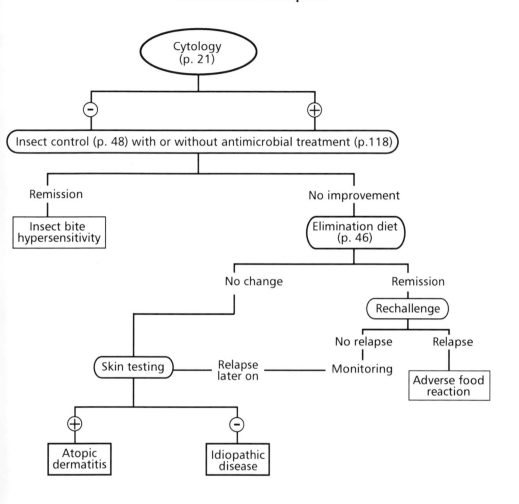

The Cat with Nodules

Key Questions

✓ How old was this patient when clinical signs were first recognized? (p. 3)

✓ How long has the disease been present and how did it progress? (p. 3)

✓ Are there other clinical signs such as sneezing, coughing, or diarrhea? (p. 7)

✓ Was the disease treated before? If so, which drugs were used and how successful was treatment? (p. 8)

Differential Diagnoses

The differential diagnoses depend primarily on two features: the number of lesions and whether draining tracts are present or not. Is there only one lesion? This increases the likelihood of neoplasia or a kerion. Or are there multiple lesions? These may be due to sterile inflammatory diseases, more aggressive neoplastic disease, or severe infection. The presence of draining tracts increases the likelihood of foreign bodies, severe bacterial or fungal infection, or sterile inflammatory disease.

In a cat with nodules, history taking and clinical examination are followed by microscopic evaluation of impression smears (if draining tracts are present) and aspirates (in any cat with nodules) (p. 21). In some patients, cytology will reveal an infectious organism or classic neoplastic cells and thus a diagnosis. In most patients, cytology will aid in further limiting the list of differential diagnoses, but a biopsy (p. 38) will be necessary to reach a diagnosis. With nodular lesions, a complete excision of one or more nodules should be performed. If draining tracts are present and/or cytology indicates possible infection, a tissue culture may be useful as well (p. 43).

The differential diagnoses for feline nodules are listed in Table 2-11.

Table 2-11
Differential Diagnoses, Commonly Affected Sites, and Recommended Diagnostic Tests in a Cat with Nodules

DISEASE	COMMONLY AFFECTED SITES	TREATMENT	PROGNOSIS
Neoplasia*	Varies with individual neoplastic diseases	Surgical excision and/or tumor specific therapy	Poor to excellent depending on the individual tumor.
Abscesses (caused by bite wounds or foreign bodies)	Fluctuating nodules most commonly around neck, shoulders, and tailbase	Surgical drainage, antibacterial treatment (p. 118)	Good
Opportunistic mycobacterial infection* (ubiquitous, facultatively pathogenic organisms such as Mycobacteria fortuitum, M. chelonei, M. smegmatis, cause lesions after traumatic implantation into subcutaneous tissue)	Nonhealing ulcerated nodules with draining tracts predominantly in the abdominal or inguinal area (Figures 2-58 and 2-59).	Wide surgical excision followed by combination antimicrobial therapy (p. 131)	Fair with appropriate surgical approach
Cryptococcosis* (uncommon infection of sometimes immunocompromised host with ubiquitous, saprophytic, yeast-like fungus Cryptococcus neoformans)	Upper respiratory, cutaneous, CNS, and ocular signs. Firm swelling over the bridge of the nose (Figure 2-60), papules, nodules, ulcers and draining tracts. Nose, lips, and claw beds maybe affected.	Antimycotic therapy with azoles and/or amphotericin B (p. 131)	Fair
Bacterial pseudomycetoma (nonbranching bacteria such as coagulase-positive Staphylococci implanted by trauma form grains of compact colonies surrounded by pyogranulomatous inflammation; rare disease)	Firm nodules with draining fistulae (Figure 2-61)	Complete surgical excision, postsurgical antibacterial treatment (p. 118)	Fair with complete excision; guarded, if this is not possible.

Table 2-11 continued

Disease	Commonly Affected Sites	Treatment	Prognosis
Eumycotic mycetoma (ubiquitous soil saprophytes cause disease through wound contamination; rare disease)	Nodules with draining tracts and scar tissue. Grains vary in size, shape, and color.	Wide surgical excision followed by antimycotic therapy (p. 131) based on in vitro susceptibility testing.	Fair to guarded depending on surgical excision.
Feline Leprosy* (presumably transmission of an incompletely characterized mycobacterium that is difficult to culture through bite wounds from rats; rare disease in veterinary dermatology)	Single or multiple, nonpainful and nonpruritic nodules on head and limbs; sometimes ulcers and fistulae are present (Figure 2-62 A and B)	Surgical excision, combination antibiotic therapy (p. 119)	Fair
Actinobacillosis* (Oral commensal aerobic *Actinobacillus lignieresii* is traumatically implanted, often through bite wounds; rare disease in veterinary dermatology)	Thick-walled abscesses of the head, mouth, and limbs discharging thick pus with soft yellow granules.	Surgical excision or drainage and long-term antibacterial therapy with streptomycin, chloramphenicol, sodium iodide or tetracyclines (p. 118, 121)	Guarded
Histoplasmosis (uncommon infection with dimorphic, saprophytic soil fungus *Histoplasma capsulatum*; very rare disease in veterinary dermatology)	Papules, nodules, ulcers, and draining tracts with concurrent anorexia, weight loss, and fever; dyspnea and ocular disease	Antimycotic therapy with azoles, possibly in combination with amphotericin B (p. 131)	Guarded to grave
Nocardiosis* (*Nocardia spp.* are soil saprophytes that cause respiratory, cutaneous, or disseminated infections; very rare disease in veterinary dermatology)	Ulcerated nodules and abscesses, often with draining tracts, on the limbs and ventral abdomen	Surgical drainage, antibacterial therapy based on in vitro susceptibility testing.	Guarded

Disease	Clinical Signs	Treatment	Prognosis
Phaeohyphomycosis* (wound contamination by ubiquitous saprophytic fungi with pigmented hyphae; very rare disease in veterinary dermatology)	Often solitary subcutaneous nodules on nose, trunk, or extremities	Wide surgical excision followed by antimycotic therapy (p. 131) based on in vitro susceptibility testing.	Guarded
Plague (infection with *Yersinia pestis* by inhalation of organism or through wound contamination or flea bites; very rare disease in veterinary dermatology) Zoonosis: Spread through transmission of infected fleas, presentation of infected killed rodents, or direct infection!	High fever, depression, anorexia, and abscesses typically on the face or limbs in the bubonic form. Septicemic and pneumonic forms also exist.	Flea control (p. 136), draining of abscesses, antibacterial therapy with tetracycline, streptomycin, or chloramphenicol (p. 118)	Fair, if recognized and treated promptly.
Sporotrichosis* (caused by ubiquitous dimorphic fungal saprophyte *Sporothrix schenkii* that infects wounds; uncommon disease in veterinary dermatology) Zoonosis: Transmission to humans through contact with an ulcerated wound easily possible!	Multiple nodules or ulcerated plaques on the head, distal limbs, tailbase (Figure 2-63). Anorexia, lethargy, fever, and depression possible concurrently	Antimycotic therapy with iodides or azoles (p. 131)	Fair
Sterile granulomatous and pyogranulomatous disease (unknown pathogenesis)	Firm, painless, nonpruritic dermal papules, plaques, and nodules typically on head and pinnae	Doxycycline / Niacinamide (p. 121), immunosuppressive therapy (p. 141), may resolve spontaneously	Fair
Sterile panniculitis (unknown pathogenesis)	Solitary nodules on ventral rump	Surgical excision	Good

Table 2-11 continued

DISEASE	COMMONLY AFFECTED SITES	TREATMENT	PROGNOSIS
Tuberculosis* (very rare in small animal dermatology; predominantly respiratory and digestive lesions)	Insidious ulcers, plaques, and nodules on head, neck, and limbs discharging yellow-green pus with unpleasant odor.	Combination antimicrobial therapy, frequent euthanasia (public health concerns).	Poor

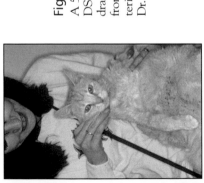

Figure 2-58
A 5-year-old castrated DSH with nodules and draining tracts resulting from atypical mycobacteria. (Courtesy of Dr. Sonya Bettenay.)

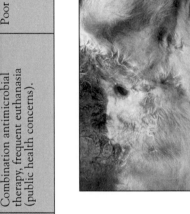

Figure 2-59
Draining tracts due to atypical mycobacteria in a 3-year-old castrated DSH.

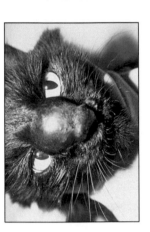

Figure 2-60
Nasal swelling caused by cryptococcosis in a 6-year-old female domestic longhair cat. (Courtesy of Dr. Thierry Olivry.)

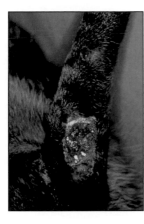

Figure 2-61
Pseudomycetoma in a Persian cat. (Courtesy of Dr. Peter Ihrke.)

Figure 2-62A
Feline leprosy in a DSH. (Courtesy of Dr. Peter Ihrke.)

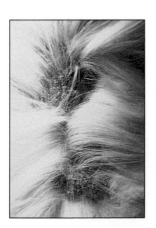

Figure 2-62B
Closeup of feline leprosy in a DSH. (Courtesy of Dr. Peter Ihrke.)

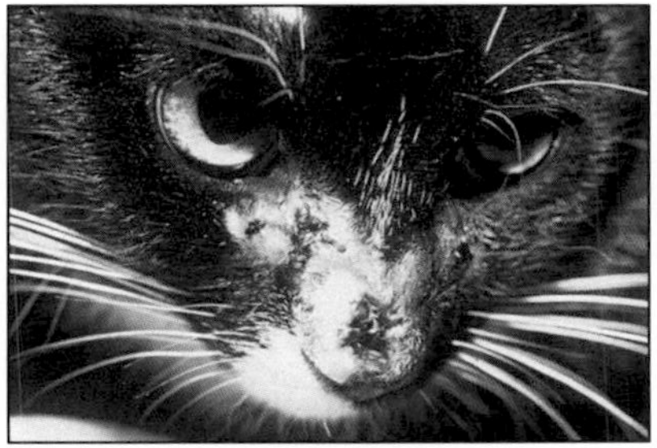

Figure 2-63
Nasal ulceration in a 2-year-old castrated DSH with sporotrichosis.

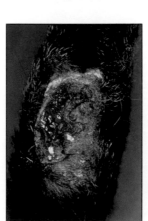

Figure 2-64
The Cat with Nodules

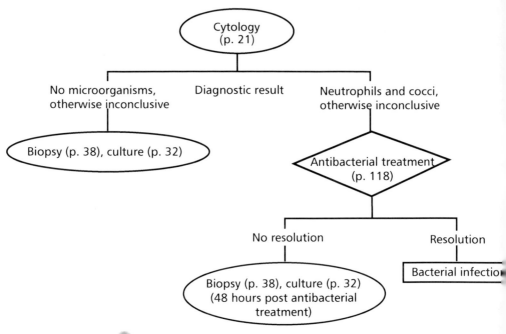

Cytology
(p. 21)

No microorganisms,
otherwise inconclusive

Diagnostic result

Neutrophils and cocci,
otherwise inconclusive

Biopsy (p. 38), culture (p. 32)

Antibacterial treatment
(p. 118)

No resolution

Resolution

Biopsy (p. 38), culture (p. 32)
(48 hours post antibacterial
treatment)

Bacterial infectio

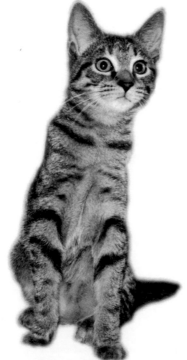

The Patient with Otitis Externa

Otitis externa may be seen with many diseases in conjunction with other clinical signs, which are helpful in the formulation of a list of differential diagnoses. This discussion is the approach to the dog with otitis externa and no other symptoms.

It is important to differentiate between predisposing, primary, and perpetuating factors in the pathogenesis of otitis externa. Predisposing factors are independent from the underlying disease and alone will not cause disease, but will facilitate the pathologic process. Conformation, including dense hair in the ear canal, a long and narrow ear canal, pendulous ears, and climate-related seasonal factors such as increased temperature and humidity are examples of predisposing factors. Complicating factors occur only after the primary pathologic process has begun, but continue to be a problem after the primary disease has been successfully identified and treated. Examples are otitis media, bacterial or fungal infections, and chronic proliferative changes due to inflammation. These complicating factors need to be treated independently. The most common primary factors are listed in Table 2-12.

Key Questions

✔ How old was this patient when clinical signs were first recognized? (p. 3)

✔ Is the disease seasonal? (p. 3)

✔ What do you feed the animal? Was a special diet used in the past? (p. 7)

✔ Are there any other animals in the household? (p. 8)

✔ Was the disease treated before? If so, which drugs were used and how successful was treatment? (p. 8)

✔ When was the last medication given? (p. 9)

Table 2-12
Differential Diagnoses, Important Clinical Clues, Recommended Diagnostic Tests, Treatment Options, and Prognosis in a Patient with Otitis Externa

DISEASE	COMMENTS	DIAGNOSTIC TESTS	TREATMENT	PROGNOSIS
Atopy* (hypersensitivity to aeroallergens such as pollens, house dust mites, or mold spores). (Figure 2-65)	In some patients a seasonal condition; unilateral otitis externa may be caused by atopy	Diagnosis based on history, physical examination, and ruling out differential diagnoses. Intradermal skin test or serum test for allergen-specific IgE (p. 42) identify offending allergens and allow formulation of immunotherapy.	Allergen-specific immunotherapy (p. 123), antihistamines (p. 125), essential fatty acids (p. 128), glucocorticoids (p. 129), topical glucocorticoids.	Good for well-being of the patient with continued management, guarded for cure.
Otodectes cynotis infestation (very common cause, particularly in young animals and cats)	Coffee grounds appearance of debris in the ear canals	Otoscopic examination. Microscopic evaluation of debris from ear swabs suspended in mineral oil; miticidal treatment trial (p. 49)	Antiparasitic agents such as ivermectin (p. 133) systemically, although many patients will respond to topical miticidal therapy	Excellent
Foreign body	Typically unilateral and of acute onset	Otoscopic examination	Removal	Excellent
Scabies (a highly contagious disease caused by Sarcoptes scabiei var. canis in dogs and Notoedres cati in cats)	Edges and lateral aspects of pinnae affected as well as (or worse than) the canal (Figure 2-66).	Superficial skin scrapings (p. 26), sarcoptes treatment trial (p. 49).	Antiparasitic agents (p. 133)	Excellent
Food adverse reaction (may or may not be allergic; commonly a reaction against a protein, rarely an additive; clinically indistinguishable from atopy)	Unilateral otitis externa maybe seen with food adverse reactions	Elimination diet (p. 46)	Avoidance, antihistamines (p. 125), essential fatty acids (p. 128), glucocorticoids (p. 129), topical glucocorticoids.	Excellent, if offending protein(s) is (are) identified and avoided; otherwise fair with continued management. Poor chance of cure.

Condition	Clinical signs	Diagnosis	Treatment	Prognosis
Hyperadrenocorticism* (spontaneous or idiopathic. The spontaneous form is an excessive production of glucocorticoids either due to a microadenoma or macroadenoma of the pituitary gland (PDH, 85%) or due to adrenocortical neoplasms in 15%)	Subtle clinical signs may be overlooked (see table 2-5). Complete response to therapy of secondary ear infection	Serum biochemistry (SAP↑↑, cholesterol ↑, ALT ↑, glucose ↑, urea ↓), hemograms (leukocytosis, neutrophilia, lymphopenia and eosinopenia), urinalysis (specific gravity ↓, cortisol:creatinine ratio ↑), radiographs (hepatomegaly, osteoporosis, mineralization of adrenal glands), low-dose dexamethasone suppression test, ACTH assays, ultrasonography (adrenal gland size ↑), ACTH stimulation test	Iatrogenic form: discontinue glucocorticoid administration. Idiopathic form: o,p -DDD (mitotane), ketoconazole for PDH (p. 131), surgical removal of affected gland for adrenocortical neoplasia	Approximately 60% of dogs with adrenal tumors were reported to survive adrenalectomy and the postoperative period. The average life expectancy was 36 months. Adrenal adenocarcinomas have a better prognosis than adenomas. The life span of dogs with PDH treated medically averaged 30 months with some dogs living longer than 10 years and others only days.
Pemphigus foliaceus* (immune-mediated skin disease characterized by intraepidermal pustule formation due to pemphigus antibodies against antigens in the intercellular connections. May be drug-induced or paraneoplastic)	Inner surface of pinnae typically worse than canals (Figure 2-67)	Cytology (p. 21), biopsy (p. 38)	Immunosuppression (p. 141)	Fair with appropriate treatment, poor for cure (except drug-induced pemphigus)
Neoplasia* (ceruminous gland adenomas and adenocarcinomas–both types in cats, the former more common in dogs)	Unilateral, older animals	Otoscopic examination	Surgical excision (vertical or complete ablation of the ear canal)	Good, if completely excised and no metastases

Table 2-12 continued

Disease	Commonly Affected Sites	Diagnostic Tests	Treatment	Prognosis
Hypothyroidism (lymphocytic thyroiditis, presumably autoimmune, or idiopathic thyroid necrosis which may be end-stage lymphocytic thyroiditis)	Subtle other clinical signs may be overlooked (see Table 2-5). Complete response to therapy of secondary ear infection	Serum biochemistry (SAP↑, cholesterol ↑, ALT ↑), hemograms (anemia), thyroid tests (free T4, total T4, free T4 by equilibrium dialysis, TSH assays, TSH stimulation test, TRH stimulation test)	Hormone replacement therapy with levothyroxine (p. 144)	Good, although not all patients stay in complete and constant remission despite adequate supplementation.
Idiopathic seborrhea* (primary keratinization defect as autosomal recessive trait with decreased epidermal cell renewal time and thus hyperproliferation of epidermis, sebaceous glands, and follicular infundibulum secondary to inflammation, endocrine disease, or nutritional deficiencies)	Excessive wax formation even with topical medication.	Biopsy (p. 38)	Ear cleaners, retinoids, corticosteroids	Fair to guarded for well-being; poor for cure

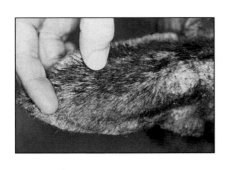

Figure 2-66
Pinnal scaling and crusting in a male Great Dane with scabies (Courtesy of Dr. Sonya Bettenay).

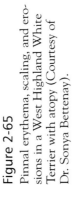

Figure 2-65
Pinnal erythema, scaling, and erosions in a West Highland White Terrier with atopy (Courtesy of Dr. Sonya Bettenay).

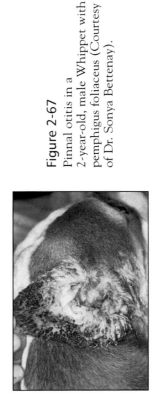

Figure 2-67
Pinnal otitis in a 2-year-old, male Whippet with pemphigus foliaceus (Courtesy of Dr. Sonya Bettenay).

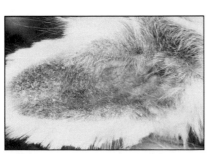

Figure 2-68
Identification of the Primary Disease in the Patient with Otitis Externa

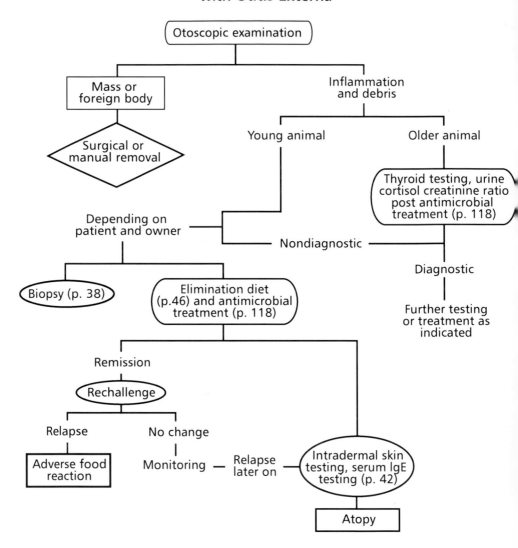

Cytology is essential in any dog or cat with otitis externa; examination must be separate in the left and right ear canals as infective microorganisms may be different from one ear to the other. In some animals, particularly in patients with chronic long-standing otitis externa and concurrent otitis media, organisms in the middle ear may differ from the those isolated in the external ear. Antimicrobial treatment in the ear canal is most effective topically and determined by cytology (p. 21) and in vitro susceptibility (p. 42 and 46). Repeat cytology examinations during treatment is essential and changes in the otic flora may necessitate changing medications.

Otitis media is best treated with systemic medication. Many dogs with chronic otitis externa and otitis media may not respond to treatment because of severe accumulation of purulent or waxy material in the ear canals. An ear flush under anesthesia may be needed followed by a new attempt of topical and concurrent systemic therapy. The tympanum may rupture prior to flushing or during flushing because in an inflamed ear the tympanum is much more fragile than normal. Frequently there are few alternatives for antimicrobial treatment in these patients. Sometimes they may have to receive potentially ototoxic topical medication. Be sure to discuss this possibility with owners before beginning therapy. Regular cytologic examinations are a precondition for successful management of patients with otitis externa. They are not specifically mentioned in Figure 2-68. Therapeutic trials and tests for primary diseases may be influenced by concurrent topical medication and thus must be planned, executed, and interpreted with care. Chronic long-standing otitis externa is extremely frustrating for patients, clients, and veterinarians, and patients may benefit from referral to a veterinary dermatologist.

Section 3

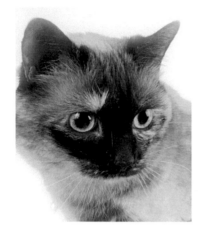

Treatments

In this section, I will summarize the most common treatment modalities, their formulations (which may vary in different parts of the world), indications, and doses. Given that detailed discussion of individual drugs, their mechanisms of action, pharmacokinetics, and protocols is beyond the scope of this text, further reading may be required. See Recommended Readings.

Drugs marked with an (✻) and a colored screen are potentially dangerous and the clinician inexperienced with these medications may consider offering referral to a veterinary specialist or seeking further advice from a colleague with more knowledge about that particular agent.

Shampoo Therapy of Various Skin Conditions

Shampoo therapy can provide effective management of dermatoses with both medical and cosmetic presenting complaints (Table 3-1). There are few adverse effects associated with shampoo therapy, although they are recognized. However, shampoo therapy is symptomatic treatment; it rarely "cures" a dermatosis.

Prescribing a shampoo involves selecting the proper shampoo for both the dermatosis and the client. Shampoo manufacturers have undertaken considerable research and development in order to produce formulations, which lather well, have an appealing smell, offer little irritation, and serve their intended purposes.

In addition to selecting the appropriate shampoo, the veterinarian's instructions will have a significant impact on the efficacy. The frequency of bathing and duration of skin contact time will influence the obtained result. A 10-minute contact time is generally recommended. This is a long time for the owner of a fidgety, shivering dog to wait and it will frequently be cut short! Techniques to improve contact time include:

✓ Take a clock into the bathing area and time 10 minutes accurately.

✓ Use the time for patting and bonding.

✓ Massage the skin for the full 10 minutes; it will usually be enjoyable for the dog and occupy both pet and owner.

✓ Take the dog outside to play ball or go for a walk with the soap still on (if climate permits).

✓ Rinse the shampoo off thoroughly for at least 5 to 10 minutes.

The frequency of shampooing will vary with severity and type of the disease process. In general, the more severe the disease, the more frequently bathing is indicated.

The major reasons for failure of shampoo therapy are

1. lack of client compliance (frequency and/or duration of application)
2. incorrect selection of shampoo for the disease process
3. shampoo irritation

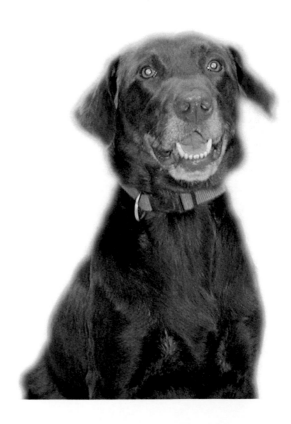

Table 3-1

Selected Shampoo Types for the Treatment of Skin Disease

Shampoo type	Comments	Indications	Frequency of administration
Chlorhexidine	Antibacterial, antifungal, not inactivated by organic matter, not irritating or drying, may be used in dogs and cats	Bacterial infections. May also be helpful in decreasing environmental contamination in patients with fungal infection	q 1-14 days
Benzoyl peroxide	Degreasing (and thus drying), keratolytic, possibly follicular flushing. In dogs with dry or normal skin, a moisturizer must be used after the shampoo! May be irritating, particularly in concentrations over 3%. Should not be used in cats!	Bacterial infections, sebaceous adenitis, demodicosis	q 7-14 days
Ethyl lactate	May be drying. Controversial efficacy in different studies	Superficial pyoderma	q 7-14 days
Iodine	Antifungal, antibacterial, virucidal, sporicidal, degreasing, but also staining and potentially irritating!	Superficial pyoderma. May also be helpful in decreasing environmental contamination in patients with fungal infection	q 7-14 days
Sulfur	Keratoplastic and keratolytic, antibacterial and mildly antifungal. Synergistic with salicylic acid	Seborrhea sicca, seborrheic dermatitis.	q 3-14 days
Salicylic acid	Keratolytic, mildly anti-inflammatory, synergistic action with sulfur	Seborrhea sicca, seborrheic dermatitis	q 3-14 days
Tar	Keratoplastic and keratolytic, antipruritic and degreasing. In dogs with dry or normal skin, it needs to be followed with a moisturizer. Not to be used in cats!	Seborrheic dermatitis, seborrhea oleosa	q 3-14 days
Colloidal oatmeal	Hydrates the stratum corneum	Pruritic skin disease, dry skin	q 2-14 days

Treatment of Bacterial Infection

✓ Antibiotics are frequently used in veterinary dermatology, because many conditions are associated with secondary bacterial infection. Dogs with chronic allergies, immune-mediated dermatoses, or endocrinopathies frequently develop secondary pyodermas that exacerbate these conditions and necessitate antibacterial treatment (Table 3-2).

✓ Not all available antibiotics are useful for skin infections so that spectrum of activity as well as pharmacology of the different antibacterial drugs has to be considered.

🗝 The overwhelming majority of skin infections in the dog and cat is caused by *Staphylococcus intermedius*. Mixed infections can involve organisms such as *Escherichia coli* or *Pseudomonas aeruginosa*, which usually develop concurrently with most patients' primary agent, *S. intermedius*.

🗝 Proper dosage and proper duration are important for the success of antibacterial therapy. Antibiotics should be given for at least 3 weeks or longer or until at least 1 week after resolution of clinical signs. Relapses are common in patients on short courses of pharmacotherapy or those receiving medications at low dosages! Deep infections may take 6 to 12 weeks to resolve.

✓ Pyodermas can, at least initially, be treated empirically. If appropriate therapy does not resolve the condition, taking a culture is indicated (p. 32).

✓ Each sample for culture and sensitivity should be accompanied by cytologic examination and culture results interpreted in light of the cytology, as growth of different microorganisms does not indicate necessarily that they are present in significant numbers in vivo.

Table 3-2
Selected Antibiotics in Small Animal Dermatology

Drug	Formulation	Comments	Adverse Effects	Indications	Dog Dose (D) Cat Dose (C)
Trimethoprim/ sulfamethoxazole	5/25 mg and 20/100 mg coated tablets, 40 mg/ 200 mg, 80 mg/400 mg, and 160 mg/800 mg tablets, 8 mg/40 mg/ml syrup.	**Not for Doberman Pinschers.** Resistance pattern varies, low in England and the United States, high in Australia	Keratoconjunctivitis sicca, drug reactions (cutaneous eruptions, polyarthritis, bone marrow suppression), hepatotoxic, gastrointestinal symptoms, fever, hypothyroidism with extended use	Infections with gram-positive bacteria. Many gram-negative organisms of the family *Enterobacteriaceae* are also susceptible (but not *Pseudomonas aeruginosa*).	15-30 mg/kg q 12 h (D, C)
Trimethoprim/ sulfadiazine	180 mg/820 mg tablets, 9 mg/41 mg/ml syrup	**Not for Doberman Pinschers.** Resistance pattern varies, low in England and the United States, high in Australia	Keratoconjunctivitis sicca, drug reactions (cutaneous eruptions, polyarthritis, bone marrow suppression), hepatotoxic, gastrointestinal symptoms, fever, hypothyroidism with extended use	Infections with gram-positive bacteria. Many gram-negative organisms of the family *Enterobacteriaceae* are also susceptible (but not *Pseudomonas aeruginosa*).	15-30 mg/kg q 12 h (D, C)
Erythromycin	250 mg and 500 mg tablets, 500 mg coated tablets, 20 mg/ml, 40 mg/ml, 80 mg/ml, 120 mg/ml syrup.	Give without food. Inexpensive! Resistance develops relatively quickly. Do not administer concurrently with terfenadine, cyclosporine, or ketaconazole	Vomiting, diarrhea, nausea	Bacterial superficial pyoderma	15 mg/kg q 8 h without food (D, C)
Lincomycin	200 and 500 mg tablets, 500 mg capsules.	Give without food. Contraindicated in rabbits, hamsters, and guinea pigs!	Vomiting, diarrhea (less common than with erythromycin)	Infections with most gram-positive cocci including *Staphylococci*. *Nocardia* and *Actinomyces* may also be susceptible.	20-30 mg/kg q 12 h without food (D, C)

Table 3-2 continued

Drug	Formulation	Comments	Adverse Effects	Indications	Dog Dose (D) Cat Dose (C)
Penicillin V	125, 250, 500 mg tablets, 25 mg/ml and 50 mg/ml oral suspension.	Not commonly used in dermatology because most strains of *Staphylococcus intermedius* are resistant to penicillin	Gastrointestinal signs with oral administration, hypersensitivity reactions	Infections with *Actinomyces*, most spirochetes and gram-positive and gram–negative cocci, which do not produce penicillinase.	10 mg/kg q 6-8 h (D, C)
Amoxicillin	500 mg, 750 mg, 1000 mg tablets, 50 mg/ml syrup.	Not commonly used in dermatology because most *Staphylococcus intermedius* strains are resistant to amoxycillin.	Vomiting, diarrhea, allergic reactions	Most organisms that cause skin disease are resistant to ampicillin and amoxycillin, thus it is rarely indicated.	10-20 mg/kg q 8 h (D, C)
Clavulanic acid/amoxycillin	12.5/50 mg, 62.5/250 mg, 125/500 mg tablets, 12.5/50 mg syrup	In vitro resistance of Staphylococci extremely low, but sensitivity in vitro not always correlating with results in vivo. May be more efficacious with q 8 h administration.	Vomiting, diarrhea, allergic reactions	Bacterial pyoderma	12.5-25 mg/kg q 8-12h (D, C)
Cloxacillin	250 mg and 500 mg capsules, 25 mg/ml solution	Effective against most gram-positive cocci	Vomiting, diarrhea, allergic reactions	Pyoderma caused by sensitive cocci	20-40 mg/kg q 8h (D, C)
Cephalexin	500 mg, 1000 mg tablets, 250 mg, 500 mg capsules, 75 mg, 300 mg, 600 mg tablets, 50 mg/ml syrup	Used commonly in veterinary dermatology	Vomiting and diarrhea; very rarely excitability, tachypnea or blood dyscrasias.	Superficial and deep bacterial pyodermas	20-30 mg/kg q 8-12h (D, C)
Cefadroxil	1000 mg tablets, 50 mg/ml syrup		Vomiting and diarrhea, very rarely tachypnea or blood dyscrasias	Superficial and deep bacterial pyodermas	20-30 mg/kg q 8-12 h (D, C)

Drug	Formulation	Comments	Side effects	Indications	Dosage
Tetracycline	250 mg, 500 mg capsules	Should not be given with amphotericin B or erythromycin. In veterinary dermatology used for immunomodulatory effects	Nausea, vomiting, discoloration of teeth in puppies and kittens, phototoxic reactions, hepatotoxicity	In combination with niacinamid used for the treatment of discoid lupus erythematosus, idiopathic onychomadesis.	250-500 mg/animal q 8 h (in combination with niacinamide at 250-500 mg/animal q 8 h) (D, C)
Doxycyline	50 mg, 100 mg, 200 mg capsules, 100 mg/ml paste, 1 mg/ml, 5 mg/ml suspension	Also used for effects on cells of the immune system and cytokine production	Nausea, vomiting, discoloration of teeth in puppies and kittens; phototoxic reactions	Bacterial superficial pyoderma, mycobacterial infections, discoid lupus erythematosus.	2.5-5 mg/kg q 24 h (if used for immune-mediated diseases, it is combined with niacinamide at 250-500 mg/animal q 8 h) (D, C)
Clindamycin	75 mg, 150 mg, 300 mg capsules	Do not give concurrently with cyclosporin, iron supplementation, and oral diabetic agents.	Skin rashes, vomiting, diarrhea.	Infections with gram-positive cocci, most anaerobic organisms, Nocardia, Actinomyces	5-10 mg/kg q 12h (D, C)
Enrofloxacin	5,7 mg, 22.7 mg, 50 mg, 68 mg, 136 mg, 150 mg tablets	Not in immature animals! Ineffective against anaerobic organisms. Resistance may occur, particularly to Pseudomonas.	Cartilage erosions in puppies, vomiting and diarrhea. Hypersensitivities and CNS signs could potentially occur. Crystalluria may occur in dehydrated animals	Infections with staphylococci, mycobacteria, most gram-negative organisms	5-20 mg/kg q 24 h (D) 5 mg/kg q 24 h (C)
Ciprofloxacin	100 mg, 250 mg , 500 mg, 750 mg coated tablets	Ineffective against anaerobe organisms. Resistance may occur, particularly to Pseudomonas.	Cartilage erosions in puppies; vomiting and diarrhea. Hypersensitivities and CNS signs could potentially occur. Crystalluria may occur in dehydrated animals	Infections with staphylococci, mycobacteria, most gram-negative organisms	5-15 mg/kg q 12 h (D, C)

Table 3-2 continued

Drug	Formulation	Comments	Adverse Effects	Indications	Dog Dose (D) Cat Dose (C)
Marbofloxacin	25-mg, 50-mg, 100-mg, 200-mg scored coated tablets	Not in immature animals! Ineffective against anaerobe organisms. Resistance may occur, particularly to *Pseudomonas*.	Cartilage erosions in puppies, vomiting and diarrhea. Hypersensitivities and CNS signs could potentially occur.	Infections with staphylococci, mycobacteria, most gram-negative organisms	2.5-5 mg/kg q 24 h without food (D, C)
Mupirocin	2% ointment	Effective against gram-positive organisms, particularly *Staphylococci*.		Localized superficial bacterial infections, feline acne.	Apply to affected areas q 12 h, prevent animal from licking area for 10 minutes (D, C)

Treatment of Pruritus

Allergen-specific Immunotherapy*

Specific immunotherapy was introduced to veterinary medicine in the1960s. Since then several studies have been undertaken to evaluate the efficacy of allergy shots in dogs and cats. Despite the use of different allergens (aqueous versus aluminum-precipitated) and different protocols, the overall success rate was comparable and varied from 45% to 60% in studies with a follow-up of 1 year or longer to 70% to 100% in studies with a shorter duration.

In specific immunotherapy, an individual is exposed to extracts of antigens to which it has shown an allergic reaction. This exposure starts at low concentrations that are increased gradually over time and after reaching a maintenance dose, are either continued indefinitely or slowly tapered.

Considerations before Beginning Allergen-specific Immunotherapy

Clinically and relevant to daily practice, several key issues need to be discussed with owners before they consider allergen-specific immunotherapy or "allergy shots".

✓ The success rate: About 20% of the patients will do extremely well and thrive with no additional therapy; 40% of the patients do well, even though occasional additional treatments such as antihistamines, fatty acids and/or antibiotics are needed. Owners are happy with the improvement achieved and consider the allergy shots worthwhile, even though therapy may be lifelong. Another 20% of patients improve, but the degree of improvement is unsatisfactory. And in 20% of the patients therapy has no influence on the disease process.

✓ The cost: This may vary depending on the country of practice, the dog's allergies, the vaccines used, and the dose rates needed. Veterinary dermatologists are a good source of information for approximate expense.

✓ The time to improvement: First improvement may be seen as early as 4 weeks into therapy and as late as 12 months after starting the allergy shots. On average, improvement is expected after between 4 and 6 months.

✓ The duration of treatment: A minority of owners may discontinue their dogs' immunotherapy after 2 years, with their pets being permanently cured and symptom free. Other dogs, however, will require lifelong therapy!

✓ The involvement: Atopic dogs are "high maintenance" and as such need constant care, most likely at least initially regular rechecks and concurrent medication. Allergy shots are not an easy way out but at this point the best of many available treatments, all of which involve long-term administration of medications of some sort.

Points to Remember if You Have Patients on Immunotherapy

✋ Glucocorticoids may be given on an occasional basis at anti-inflammatory dosage levels without interfering with therapy.

✓ Antihistamines, fatty acids, and antimicrobials do not interfere with immunotherapy so that they may be, and often are, used concurrently.

🔑 If the condition of patients receiving allergy shots suddenly deteriorates, always evaluate for infection. Yeast and bacteria are common complicating factors secondary to these allergies, which can cause dramatic increases in pruritus. Cytology (p. 21) will identify cocci, rods, yeasts and inflammatory cells and thereby guide antimicrobial therapy.

✓ If no infection is detected, antihistamines or glucocorticoids can be used to regulate the patient's pruritus.

✓ If there is a regular increase in pruritus after the injection, the dose and frequency may need to be adjusted. Decreased doses may be helpful.

✓ If there is a regular increase in pruritus before the injection that is greatly improved by the injection of allergen extract, the time interval between the injections is probably too long and needs to be shortened. The dose may also be decreased in some of these patients without decreased efficacy.

✔ If there is no response to allergen-specific immunotherapy after 4 to 6 months, I recommend that you contact your nearest veterinary dermatologist for advice while there is still sufficient vaccine left to change the dose and frequency of the injections by adjusting them to the needs of that particular patient. Many patients need an approach suiting their particular requirements and the help of a veterinarian experienced in immunotherapy may be of great benefit.

I sincerely believe that allergen-specific immunotherapy is currently the best available treatment for canine atopic dermatitis, but it will only be successful in most atopic animals if owners and veterinarians have realistic expectations and are prepared to put in significant effort over the period that sometimes extends over many months. Only then will maximal benefit be achieved! In as much as the first months on immunotherapy may be draining for owner and veterinarian, consider offering referral to a veterinary dermatologist, particularly if you are not experienced in this therapy.

Antihistamines

✔ Antihistamines are useful adjunctive agents in the management of pruritic patients. The classical antihistamines act by blocking H1-receptors. First-generation antihistamines also have an anticholinergic, sedative, and local anaesthetic effect. Second-generation antihistamines penetrate less through the blood brain barrier or have a low affinity for the brain compared with the action on peripheral H1-receptors. Thus they are effective yet produce less sedation (Table 3-3).

✔ The advantage of antihistamines is the rare occurrence of adverse effects. Drowsiness is the most common finding and may decrease after 2 to 3 days of therapy. Thus, it may be worthwhile continuing treatment for several days before final evaluation. Less common are gastrointestinal signs. Acute poisoning following an overdose is characterized by CNS hyperexcitability. Due to the anticholinergic properties of terfenadine and cyproheptadine, these drugs should not be used in patients with severe cardiovascular disease, since they may cause hypertension.

✔ The necessity of frequent administration (two to three times daily) and the high cost of some antihistamines limit their long-term use in many patients, especially larger dogs.

✔ A further shortcoming in dogs is the relatively low success rate, which varies between 5% and 30%, depending on dosage and drug used.

☞ Cats are much more likely to respond to antihistamines than dogs. However, administering oral medication on a long-term basis may be challenging in this species.

✔ If a patient responds to antihistamine therapy and the owner is willing to maintain the animal on it, antihistamines represent safe long-term treatment that is preferable to glucocorticoids!

✔ Antihistamines in humans are not used to treat present symptoms but to prevent onset of symptoms. Thus, administration should not be intermittent assuming the same holds true in animals.

✋ The potential success rate can be increased by trying several different antihistamines sequentially because patients may be responsive to one antihistamine but not to another.

✋ Antihistamines have been reported to be effective in lowering the corticosteroid dose, even if they did not help the animal as a single therapeutic agent.

✔ Because the withdrawal time of antihistamines before an intradermal skin test is much shorter than that of glucocorticoids, they can be used to relieve pruritus during the preparation time where the latter are contraindicated.

Selected Antihistamines Used in the Treatment of Small Animal Hypersensitivities

Drug	Formulation	Comments	Dog Dose (D), Cat Dose (C)
Dexchlorpheniramine	2 mg tablets, 6 mg tablets	Inexpensive, potentially sedating	2-6 mg q 8-12 h (D), 2 mg q 8-12 h (C)
Chlorpheniramine	4 mg tablets	Inexpensive, potentially sedating	2-12 mg q 12 h (D) 2-4 mg q 12 h (C)
Cyproheptadine	4 mg tablets	Inexpensive, potentially sedating	2-8 mg q 8-12 h (D) 2-4 mg q 12 h (C)
Promethazine	10 mg, 25 mg coated tablets	Sedating	1-2 mg/kg q 12 h (D, C)
Hydroxyzine	10 mg, 25 mg, 50 mg capsules	Also inhibits mast cell degranulation, and is tricyclic antidepressant and teratogenic!!	2 mg/kg q 8-12 h (D, C)
Loratidine	10 mg tablet, 1 mg/ml syrup		5-20 m q 12-24 h (D) 5 mg q 12-24 h (C)
Cetirizine	10 mg coated tablets, 1 mg/ml syrup	Inhibits exocytosis of eosinophils in humans	5-20 mg q 12-24 h (D) 5 mg q 12-24 h (C)
Clemastine	1 mg tablets, 0.05 mg/ml syrup	Enhances cholinergic activity of other antihistamines as these drugs are metabolized by same enzyme system in liver and concurrent administration may increase serum levels significantly.	0.5-1 mg q 12 h (D)
Terfenadine	60 mg, 120 mg tablets, 6 mg/ml suspension	Do not give concurrently with ketoconazole, cyclosporine, astemizol, or erythromycin as these drugs are metabolized by same enzyme system in liver and concurrent administration may increase serum levels significantly.	30-60 mg q 12 h (D)
Amitryptilline	10 mg, 25 mg tablets		1 mg/kg q 12 h (D, C)
Astemizol	10 mg tablets, 2 mg/ml suspension	Do not administer concurrently with ketoconazol, itraconazol, cyclosporine, erythromycin, or terfenadine.	0.25 mg/kg q 24 h (D, C)
Trimeprazine	2.5-10 mg, 5 mg tablets		2.5-10 mg q 8-12 h (D)
Azatidine	1 mg tablets, 0.5 mg/5 ml syrup		0.5-2mg q 12 h (D) 0.5 mg q 12 h (C)
Foxofenachin	60 mg , 120 mg, 180 mg coated tablets	Do not administer concurrently with ketoconazol, itraconazol, erythromycin, cyclosporine, or terfenadine	30-120 mg q 12 h (D)

Essential Fatty Acids

✓ Essential fatty acids (EFAs) are important for epidermal barrier function, as components of cell membranes, and as the precursors of inflammatory mediators.

✓ Supplementation with specific EFAs, especially linoleic acid (in sunflower and safflower oil), gamma-linolenic acid (in evening primrose oil) and eicosapentanoic acid (in cold water marine fish oil), can have anti-inflammatory effects. Linoleic acid is needed for maintenance of stratum corneum barrier function, limits transepidermal water loss and is thus better suited for the treatment of scaling (Table 3-4).

✓ Success rate of EFA therapy is relatively low in dogs, higher in cats.

✓ It may take several weeks of supplementation until clinical effects become evident.

✓ In essence, EFA supplementation decreases production of inflammatory prostaglandins and leukotrienes in favor of an increased production of noninflammatory or antiinflammatory prostaglandins and leukotrienes.

✓ Adjunctive therapy with essential fatty acids can be beneficial in a patient with allergies.

🖐 Fatty acids have been reported to be effective in lowering the corticosteroid dose, even if they did not help the animal as a single therapeutic agent.

🖐 Start with a small dose to avoid possible diarrhea and gradually increase the dose.

✓ Ideal doses and w-6/w-3 ratios are a subject of continuing active research.

Table 3-4
Essential Fatty Acids and Their Doses

Essential Fatty Acid	Dose
Eicosapentaenoic acid	20 mg/kg q 24 h
Linoleic acid	20-50 mg/kg q 24 h

Glucocorticoids

✓ Glucocorticoids are very commonly used in the treatment of skin conditions (Table 3-5).

✓ At anti-inflammatory dosage, they decrease inflammatory cell activity and migration.

✓ Corticosteroids are effective in most patients with atopic disease and resolve the symptoms at least initially on reasonably low dosages. Flea-allergic animals will also often respond to these drugs, although typically at slightly higher dosages.

✓ Glucocorticosteroids can be considered the treatment of choice in animals with a mild seasonal pruritus of 1 to 2 months duration that is controlled with anti-inflammatory dosages (<1 mg/kg) of prednisolone every other day.

✓ Every other day therapy is definitively preferred over daily drug administration because as it is thought to lower the chances of iatrogenic hyperadrenocorticism.

✓ I use prednisolone at anti-inflammatory doses for severely affected dogs after skin testing and short term to break the itch-scratch cycle. However, the need to increase the dosage over time to control the clinical signs in most of these patients, combined with the potentially severe long-term side effects make glucocorticoids a poor long-term choice for atopic patients.

✓ Adverse effects include polyuria, polydipsia, polyphagia, increased susceptibility to infection, and other well-known symptoms of iatrogenic hyperadrenocorticism. The most commonly encountered infections affect the urinary tract, skin, and lungs.

✓ Drugs should always be tapered to the lowest effective dose.

☞ Frequently, the dose necessary to control clinical signs can be decreased when adjunctive therapy is used. Fatty acids and antihistamines have been reported to be effective in lowering the corticosteroid dose, even if they did not help the animal as a single therapeutic agent. Regular topical therapy (e.g., shampoos) may be another means of decreasing the need for systemic glucocorticoids.

☞ I recommend to the owners of my atopic patients treated with glucocorticoids the lowest possible dose, on which the animal is mildly itchy but not uncomfortable. If no pruritus is present, the dose used is too high.

☞ The glucocorticoid dose needed with individual patients often varies seasonally.

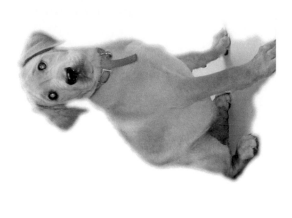

Table 3-5
Selected Glucocorticoids and Their Dosage

Drug	Formulation	Starting Dose	Dog Dose (D) / Cat Dose (C)
Prednisone	1 mg, 5 mg, 20 mg, 50 mg tablets		0.5-1 mg/kg q 24-48 h (D) 1-2 mg/kg q 24-48 h (C)
Prednisolone	1 mg, 5 mg, 20 mg, 25 mg, 50 mg tablets		0.5-1 mg/kg q 24-48 h (D) 1-2 mg/kg q 24-48 h (C)
Methylprednisolone	2 mg, 4 mg, 16 mg, 32 mg, 100 mg tablets, 20 mg/ml, 40 mg/ml Met. acetate		0.4-0.8 mg/kg q 24-48 h orally (D), intramuscularly
Dexamethasone	0.5, 1.5, 4 mg tablets, 2 mg/ml, 4 mg/ml		0.05-0.1 mg/kg q 48-72 h orally (D), 0.2-0.5 mg/ intramuscularly (D); 0.1-0.25 mg/(C),
Triamcinolone	2 mg, 4 mg, 8 mg tablets, 3 mg/ml, 10 mg/ml, 40 mg/ml		0.05-0.1 mg/kg q 48-72 h orally (D); 0.1-0.2 mg/kg IM or subcutaneously SC (D,C)

Treatment of Fungal Infections

Antimycotic agents (Table 3-6) are used after fungal infection is diagnosed by positive fluorescence under Wood's lamp (p. 30), by fungal culture (p. 32) and/or biopsy (p. 38). Ideally, treatment is continued beyond cytologic resolution (*Malassezia* spp.) or until a negative culture confirms remission (dermatophytes and systemic fungi) which is approximately 2 weeks past a negative culture and 4 weeks past cytologic resolution.

Table 3-6
Systemic Antimycotic Agents

DRUG	FORMULATION	COMMENTS	INDICATIONS	SIDE EFFECTS	DOG DOSE (D) CAT DOSE (C)
Griseofulvin	125 mg and 500 mg tablets	Administered with fatty meal	Dermatophytosis	Teratogenic! Vomiting, diarrhea, idiosyncratic bone marrow suppression	Microsize crystal form: 25-60 mg/kg q 12 h, ultramicrosize Gris-PEG 2.5-10 mg/kg q 12 h (D,C)
Ketoconazole	200 mg tablet	Administer with food! Increases blood levels of cyclosporin, phenytoin, and some antihistamines. Rifampin may decrease ketoconazole serum levels. With high-dose therapy, a slow increase over several days may minimize adverse effects.	*Malassezia*-related infections, dermatophytosis, blastomycosis, cryptococcosis, coccidioidomycosis, sporotrichosis, nocardiosis, hyperadrenocorticism	Anorexia, nausea (quite common), vomiting, diarrhea, cholangiohepatitis	2.5-10 mg/kg q 12 h for *Malassezia* infection (D, C), 10 mg/kg q 12 h for dermatophytosis (D,C), up to 20 mg/kg q 12 h for systemic mycoses (D, C), and hyperadrenocorticism (D)
Itraconazole	100 mg capsule	Administer with food! If given concurrently with cyclosporin, some antihistamines, phenytoin, or oral antidiabetic agents, the drug doses may have to be decreased. Rifampin may decrease itraconazole serum levels.	*Malassezia* and *Candida* infections, dermatophytoses, systemic mycoses	Anorexia, nausea, hepatotoxicity	5-10 mg/kg q 12-24 h (D,C)
Potassium iodide		Give with food	Sporotrichosis	Vomiting, diarrhea, depression, anorexia, hypothermia, cardiovascular failure in cats; ocular and nasal discharge, scaling and dry coat in dogs.	40 mg/kg q 12 h (D); 20 mg/kg q 12-24 h (C)

Table 3-6 continued

Drug	Formulation	Comments	Indications	Side Effects	Dog Dose (D) Cat Dose (C)
Terbinafine	250 mg tablet	Fairly new and costly drug at time of writing, limited promising information available.	Dermatophytosis	Vomiting	10-30 mg/kg q 24 h for 2-4 weeks (D,C)
Fluconazole	50-mg, 100-mg, 150-mg, 200-mg capsules	Penetrates into central nervous system (CNS) and saliva well. Dose needs to be decreased in patients with renal insufficiency. Rifampin may decrease fluconazole serum levels. Increases blood levels of cyclosporine, phenytoin and some antihistamines.	Blastomycosis, histoplasmosis, cryptococcosis, oral candidiasis	Vomiting, diarrhea, nausea, hepatotoxicity	2.5-5 mg/kg q 12 h (D); 2.5-10 mg/kg q 12 h (C)
Amphotericin B*	50-mg dry substance/bottle	Relatively toxic, thus treatment is dangerous and referral may be considered. Incompatible with saline and lactated Ringer's solution and other drugs	In combination with ketoconazole for blastomycosis, histoplasmosis, coccidiomycosis and sporotrichosis, in combination with flucytosine for cryptococcosis and candidiasis	Nephrotoxicity, anemia, phlebitis, hypokalemia	0.5 mg/kg IV in 5% dextrose every other day (D), 0.15 mg/kg IV in 5% dextrose every other day (C). Safer is subcutaneous administration of 0.5 mg/kg, amphotericin is in 400 ml of 0.45% saline containing 2.5% dextrose q 3-4 d's to a total cumulative dose of 10-25 mg/kg.

Ectoparasiticidal Agents

When treating patients with ectoparasites, environment and contact animals have to be considered as well. Environmental contamination is significant with fleas and chiggers (*Trombicula*, *Neotrombicula*, *Walchia*) and possibly with *Cheyletiella*. Contact animals must be treated for all ectoparasites except *Demodex* and chiggers, but, if dogs are affected with scabies, cats may not have to be treated and vice versa (Table 3-7)

Table 3-7

Selected Ectoparasiticidal Agents in Small Animal Dermatology

DRUG	FORMULATION	COMMENTS	INDICATIONS	SIDE EFFECTS	DOG DOSE (D) CAT DOSE (C)
Ivermectin	10 mg/kg bovine injectable solution (often given orally to small animals), 10 mg/ml equine oral solution	Idiosyncratic toxicities most common in Collies and Old English Sheepdogs, but also possible in other breeds. Gradual dose increase from 50 μg/kg on day 1 to 100 μg on day 2, 150 μg on day 3, 200 μg on day 4 and 300 μg on day 5 to identify sensitive patients before severe adverse effects occur.	Heartworm prevention. Oral and subcutaneous administration: Canine and feline scabies, *Otodectes cynotis* infestations, demodicosis, cheyletiellosis, lice Topical administration: Canine scabies	Lethargy, ataxia, tremors, mydriasis, coma, respiratory arrest	Heartworm prevention at 6 μg/kg monthly. Oral and subcutaneous administration (with gradual increase from 50 to 300 μ within 4 days): 300 μg/kg daily for demodicosis until 8 weeks after the first negative skin scraping, four administrations 1 week apart for all other ectoparasites. (D, C) Topical administration: Ivermectin pour-on for cattle administered at 500 mg/kg (0.1 ml/kg) applied along the dorsal midline twice 2 weeks apart was reported to be effective for canine scabies.

133

Table 3-7 continued

Drug	Formulation	Comments	Indications	Side effects	Dog Dose (D) Cat Dose (C)
Milbemycin oxime	2.3 mg, 5.75 mg, 11.5 mg and 23 mg tablets	Fairly costly	Heartworm prevention, scabies, demodicosis	Very safe drug	Heartworm prevention: 1 mg/kg monthly. Scabies: 2 mg/kg twice weekly for 4 weeks. Demodicosis: 2 mg/kg daily until 8 weeks after the first negative skin scraping for demodicosis. (D, C)
Lufenuron	45 mg, 90 mg, 204.9 mg, 409.8 mg tablets (dogs), 135 mg, 270 mg suspension (cats).	All household animals need to be on lufenuron for effective treatment. Breaks life cycle, no significant adulticidal activity.	Flea infestation	Very safe drug	10-15 mg/kg once monthly orally with food (D, C) or injectable every 6 months (C).
Amitraz	10.6 ml, 50 ml concentrate	Animal must not get wet in between rinses. Animals should not be rinsed when wet. Asthmatic people should not perform the rinse.	Canine demodicosis, cheyletiellosis, scabies and *Otodectes cynotis* infestation	Sedation, pruritus, hypothermia, hyperglycemia, hypotension	Mix 10.6 ml in 2 gal of water (D) and rinse q 7-14 days. Continue for 8 weeks (D) after the first-negative scraping.
Lyme sulfur	97.8% sulfurated lime solution	Safe for even puppies and kittens	Cheyletiellosis, scabies, *Otodectes cynotis* infestation. Feline demodicosis	Very safe drug	Dilute 1 part to 32 parts water, apply as rinse or dip weekly for 4 weeks (D, C)

Drug	Formulation	Comments	Indications	Side effects	Dosage
Fipronil	0.29% spray in 100 and 250 ml bottles, 9.7% solution (0.5 ml, 0.67 ml, 1.34 ml, 2.68 ml)	Spray more effective than spot-on formulation, but strong smell unavoidable during application. For highest efficacy, animals may be shampooed 48 hours before application, but not any sooner; exposure to water does not interfere with efficacy.	Flea-bite hypersensitivity, ticks, possibly scabies and cheyletiellosis	Temporary irritation at site of application, rare hypersensitivities. Contraindicated in rabbits	Spray: 4-6 ml/kg q 2-12 weeks (8-12 pumps using the 100 ml bottle, 2-4 pumps using the 250-ml bottle). (D, C) Spot-on: Apply once monthly
Selamectin	15 mg, 30 mg, 45 mg, 60 mg, 120 mg, and 240 mg tubes.	Cosmetically appealing, disperses quickly. Too early to comment further at time of writing	Flea-bite hypersensitivity, Otodectes cynotis infestation, scabies, heartworm prevention, roundworm, and hookworm infestations	Focal alopecia (reversible)	6-12 mg/kg monthly as a spot-on. (D, C)
Imidacloprid	9.1% solution (0.4 ml, 0.8 ml, 1 ml, 2.5 ml, 4 ml tubes)	Frequent shampoo therapy or water exposure will significantly decrease efficacy. Solvent may discolor lacquer on furniture.	Flea-bite hypersensitivity	Focal alopecia	0.4 ml (C)< 4 kg, 0.8 ml (C) > 4 kg. 0.4 ml (D) > 5 kg, 1 ml (D) 5-10 kg, 2.5 ml (D) 10 – 25 kg, 4 ml (D) > 25 kg
Pyrethrin	Sprays and powders at 0.05-0.2%	Repellent as well as adulticide. Low toxicity potential, salivation in cats	Flea-bite hypersensitivity	Ptyalism, tremors, ataxia, vomiting, depression, hyperaesthesia, seizures, dyspnea	Use q 24-72 h (D, C)
Permethrin	Sprays, spot-ons and shampoos at 0.2-2%	Repellent as well as adulticide. Low toxicity in dogs. Not to be used in cats!	Canine flea-bite hypersensitivity	Ptyalism, tremors, ataxia, vomiting, depression, hyperaesthesia, seizures, dyspnea	Use q 3-10 days (D)

Insect Control Trials and Individual Management of Patients with Flea-bite Hypersensitivity

Flea control trials

✓ Treatment recommendations will vary significantly with individual situations. Confirmed flea-bite hypersensitivity, suspected flea-bite hypersensitivity, or pets that show no sign of discomfort, but have some fleas, are treated very differently.

✓ Reasonably safe and effective products are available (Table 3-7). As veterinarians, we are in the best position to advise clients on a flea-control program tailored to their specific needs that considers their personality and life style as well as their pet's little peculiarities.

⚓ A major reason for failure of flea control programs is owner compliance. They are either unwilling, not educated properly, too careless, or simply not physically able to do what we ask them to do for whatever reason. Choosing the right protocol and educating owners properly, taking the time and possibly using nursing staff, brochures, and message boards will greatly increase your chance of success.

✋ With all topical products, the first application should be administered in the clinic by the veterinarian or the veterinary technician/nurse to demonstrate the correct procedure to the owner.

✓ Another reason for failure may be resistance of the organism to the products used. Resistance will always develop to any product, the question is thus not if, but rather when. In essence, we speed up evolution and create resistant fleas by putting pressure on the population when using products for flea control. However, there are ways to delay this development of resistance. The first possibility is to combine different flea products, as it is much less likely that an individual flea gets resistant to two drugs at the same time. This approach is called integrated flea control and is becoming more popular all over the world. The second possibility is to switch products quickly when signs of resistance occur and kill the resistant flea with another effective product before it has time to multiply in big numbers.

✓ **Suspected flea-bite hypersensitivity:** Aggressive flea control is needed for 4 to 6 weeks. If there is no improvement, we most likely do not deal with flea-bite hypersensitivity. With significant improvement or remission, we established a diagnosis and need to discuss long-term strategies with that particular owner. In such a trial, we usually recommend the frequent use of an adulticide in combination with an insect growth regulator in the environment to quickly lower the flea pressure (Tables 3-8 and 3-9).

✓ **Confirmed flea-bite hypersensitivity:** Ideally, we recommend an insect growth regulator/insect development inhibitor on a permanent basis (systemically, topically or in the environment) and an adulticide as needed (Tables 3-8 and 3-9). The second option is an adulticide only, in which case we need to switch products very quickly at the first sign of resistance. However, as adulticides are tapered slowly to identify the longest possible interval in between applications, recurrences may indicate insufficient frequency of application rather than resistance.

✓ **No flea-bite hypersensitivity present:** In these cases, we do not recommend flea control because permanent flea exposure may be less likely to induce flea-bite hypersensitivity than off-and-on flea control by an owner who is not pressed into compliance by an itchy pet. If the client does want to start some sort of flea control, insect growth regulators or development inhibitors are recommended.

Mosquito-bite trial

The safest and most thorough mosquito-bite trial in cats with papules and crusted papules on nose, pinnae or foot pads is to keep the patient indoors for 2 weeks. When there is no exposure to mosquitoes, the disease regresses rapidly. However, in cats used to outdoors this option may not be viable. Alternatively, exposure is decreased when outdoor activities are limited and cats are trained to come in before dawn by feeding them in the late afternoon. In addition, a mosquito repellent safe for use in cats such as pyrethrin spray may be applied by wetting a cloth and wiping the feet and head daily before the cat goes out.

Table 3-8
Administration, Advantages, and Disadvantages of Selected Flea Control Products

DRUG	ADMINISTRATION	ADVANTAGES	DISADVANTAGES	COMMENTS
Insect growth regulators/development inhibitors				
Fenoxycarb	Indoors: spray q 12 m. Outdoors: Spot treatment of allergic pet's favorite spots q 6-12 m in dry environments.	Comparatively safe and effective, rapid onset of action	Work-intensive	Foggers are more convenient but do not cover more than 2 rooms/can. The insecticide stays on shelves and furniture, but areas underneath furniture are not covered! Sprays are less convenient and more work-intensive, but insecticide is deposited only where needed. Use in all rooms with pet access! Carpeted areas, crevices, and corners as well as areas underneath furniture are most important. Indicated with frequent visiting animals not on flea control as well as at the start of an insect-control trial.
Lufenuron	10-15 mg/kg q 30 d orally (D), 25-50 mg/kg SC q 6 m (C).	Convenient, safest environmentally	Expensive in multi-pet households, lag period of several weeks to months.	Indicated in house-holds with few pets and no visits from animals without thorough flea control.
Methoprene or Pyriproxifen	Indoor spray q 6 m	Comparatively safe and effective, rapid onset of action.	Work-intensive	Foggers are more convenient, but do not cover more than 2 rooms/can. The insecticide stays on shelves and furniture, but areas underneath furniture are not covered! Sprays are less convenient and more work-intensive, but insecticide is deposited only where needed. Use in all rooms with pet access! Carpeted areas, crevices, and corners, as well as areas underneath furniture most important. Indicated with frequent visiting animals not on flea control as well as at the start of an insect control trial.

Adulticides

Fipronil	0.29 g/100 ml, 10-15 mg/kg as a spray distributed over the whole body q 2-8 week, spot-on q 2-8 week	Water-proof (but not shampoo proof!), convenient, because used only every 2-4 weeks	No repelling action, expensive in large animals, viable egg production possible.	Spray needs to be applied carefully, covering the animal's whole body. Spot-on formulation easier to apply, but less effective. Administer outdoors or in well-ventilated area due to strong smell during first minutes. Shampoo only 2 days before new application.
Imidacloprid	100 mg/ml	Convenient, because used only every 2-4 weeks, easy to apply	Not water proof, no repelling viable egg production possible.	Shampoo only 2 days before new application. Swimming or roaming in rainy weather not recommended.
Nitenpyram	Tablets q 1-2 d or as needed	Convenient, rapid onset of action, safe	Flea needs to bite animal to die, only effective for less than one day	May be given daily with no adverse effects. Particularly useful for prophylactic administration in animals on lufenuron directly before anticipated exposure in shows or visits.
Pyrethrin		Repels insects, quick knock-out	Work-intensive, rare but possible toxicities, depending on product and patient; daily-to-monthly application	Soak animal with sprays (pressure pump sprays may be useful for bigger or long-haired dogs).

Table 3-8 continued

Drug	Administration	Advantages	Disadvantages	Comments
Permethrin	744 mg in 1 ml as a spot-on for dogs <15 kg, 1488 mg in 2 ml for dogs >15 kg. Do not use in cats.	Repelling action, quick knock-out.	Work-intensive, rare but possible toxicities, depending on product and patient; daily-to-monthly application	Soak animal with sprays (pressure pump sprays may be useful for bigger or long-haired dogs).
Selamectin	6-12 mg/kg monthly as a spot-on	Easy to use, cosmetically appealing, safe	Too new to comment at time of writing	Too new to comment at time of writing.

Table 3-9
Application of Selected Flea Products in Patients with Confirmed versus Suspected Flea-bite Hypersensitivity

Drug	Confirmed Flea-bite Hypersensitivity*	Suspected Flea-bite Hypersensitivity
Fipronil spot-on	q 2-4 weeks	Not used for insect control trials
Fipronil spray	q 4 -12 weeks	q 7-14 d for 4-6 weeks*
Imidacloprid spot-on	q 4 weeks	q 7-14 d for 4-6 weeks*
Nitenpyram	In addition to lufenuron, when patient shows clinical signs or before suspected exposure	q 1-2 d for 4-6 weeks*
Permethrin spot-on	q 4 weeks	Not used for insect control trials
Permethrin spray	Varying depending on individual product up to q 7-14 d	Varying depending on individual product up to q 2-3 d for 4-6 weeks*
Pyrethrin spray	Varying depending on individual product up to q 7-14 d	Varying depending on individual product up to q 2-3 d for 4-6 weeks*
Selamectin	q 4 week	q 14 d for 4-6 weels*

* In any flea control trial adulticides are combined with an insect growth regulator used in the environment at the beginning of the trial.

Immunosuppressive Therapy

💣 Before you think about immunosuppressive therapy you must be sure about your diagnosis. It can be very dangerous for your patient to start immunosuppressive drugs based only on history and clinical examination as a confirmation of the diagnosis of immune-mediated skin disease. If the animal has an infectious disease (fungal, bacterial, or parasitic), it can rapidly deteriorate and even die. There is no place for trial therapy in immune-mediated disease (except in the case of a patient facing euthanasia otherwise).

✋ Patients with immune-mediated skin disease commonly have secondary infections that need to be identified and treated. In patients with mild-to-moderate disease, I start antimicrobial therapy 3 weeks before immunosuppressive therapy to evaluate how many of the clinical signs are due to the infection and how many are due to the immune-mediated disease. In cases of severe clinical disease, however, treatment of infection and of the immune-mediated disease should be started concurrently.

🔑 It is impossible to give you a good general purpose recipe for immunosuppression. Every dog or cat reacts differently to each of the drugs mentioned later in this section and you have to individualize treatment for each patient. Immunosuppression is a technique requiring instinct, sensitivity, and experience as well as theoretic knowledge that is beyond the scope of this text. There are, however, certain generalizations as well as certain starting dosages and ranges.

✔ Probably the best way is to start using one preferred drug, then, if your approach fails, refer the patient and learn from the way the specialist treats it. After you are familiar with that new drug, you add another one to your repertoire and use both of them and so on.

✔ The doses mentioned in Table 3-10 are starting doses that are tapered as soon as possible to the smallest effective dose.

✓ Taper the drug once the patient is in clinical remission or if adverse effects are intolerable. In a patient with severe adverse effects and concurrent clinical signs of active disease, new drugs need to be added at the same time.

💣✳ Monitoring, as described in Table 3-10, is essential. I only compromise on monitoring standards because of financial considerations in patients facing euthanasia otherwise!

✓ Some dogs will have seasonal relapses. This mechanism is currently not understood. If a well-controlled patient suddenly seems to relapse, always check for demodicosis and fungal or bacterial infections first. Rather than a flare-up of the immune-mediated disease you may be encountering a problem secondary to your treatment. These patients are immunosuppressed and thus easily may be affected by infectious diseases! Increasing the dose of the immunosuppressive drug may not always be a good idea.

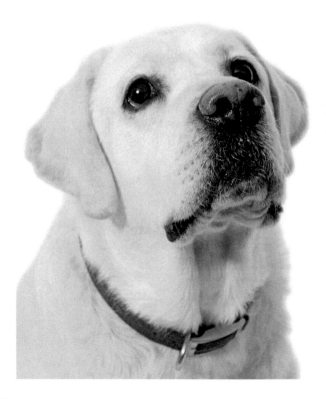

Table 3-10
Drugs Used in Immunosuppressive Therapy

DRUG	FORMULATION	COMMENTS	ADVERSE EFFECTS	DOSE: Dog Dose (D) / Cat Dose (C)	MONITORING
Prednisone/ Prednisolone	5 mg, 20 mg, 25 mg, 50 mg tablets	Rapid onset of action, inexpensive, response rate approximately 50%, high rate of adverse effects	Polyuria, polydipsia, polyphagia, lethargy, infections, muscle wasting, panting, exercise intolerance, calcinosis cutis	1-2 mg/kg q 12 h (D), 3-4 mg/kg q 12 h (C)	Urinalysis and urine cultures q 6 mo, possibly biochemistry panels and ACTH stimulation tests q 6-12 mo
Azathioprine*	25 mg tablets, 50 mg tablets	Lag period of several weeks in dogs. Should not be used in cats!!! Further reading is recommended before using this drug.	Vomiting, diarrhea (less common, if administered divided into 2 daily doses), bone marrow suppression, idiosyncratic hepatotoxicity (possibly peracute)	2 mg/kg or 50 mg/m2 q 24 h (D)	Complete blood counts at 0, 1, 2, 4, 8, 12 wk and then every 3-6 mo, possibly serum biochemistry concurrently, particularly during the first 1-2 mo.
Chlorambucil*	2 mg, 5 mg tablets	Long lag period (4-8 wk). Safest immunosuppressive agent, may be used in cats. Further reading is recommended before using this drug.	Vomiting, diarrhea, bone marrow suppression.	0.1-0.2 mg/kg q 24 h (D, C)	Complete blood counts at 0, 1, 2, 4, 8, 12 wk and then every 3-6 mo
Aurothioglucose*	50 mg/ml suspension	Long lag period (6-12 wk). May be used in cats. Some animals go into complete remission and cessation of therapy may be possible. Further reading is recommended before using this drug.	Bone marrow suppression, occasional cutaneous eruptions and proteinuria	1 mg/kg q 7 d IM (D,C) after a test dose of 1 mg/animal. Tapering to q 2 wk, 3 wk, 4 wk after remission achieved	Complete blood counts and urinalysis at 0, 1, 2, 4, 8, 12 wk and then every 3-6 mo. Serum biochemistry monthly initially, then every 3-6 mo.

Treatment of Alopecia due to Hormonal Diseases and Follicular Dysplasia (Table 3-11)

Table 3-11

Selected Drugs Used in the Treatment of Endocrine Disorders with Cutaneous Symptoms

Drug	Dose	Dog Dose (D) Cat Dose (C)	Indications	Adverse Effects
o,p'-DDD* (mitotane)		25 mg/kg q 12 h during induction (5-14 d), same dose q 12 h on 2 consecutive days of each week as maintenance. Length of induction determined by water intake, food intake, and ACTH stimulation test. (D, C)	Idiopathic hyperadrenocorticism, adrenal sex hormone imbalance (I do not recommend the drug for this latter disease). Further reading is recommended prior to using this drug.	Lethargy, ataxia, vomiting, diarrhea, anorexia.
Levothyroxine		20 μg/kg q 12 h. If patient condition is well controlled, medication may be changed to once daily at double dose. (D, C)	Hypothyroidism	Polydipsia, polyuria, nervousness, aggressiveness, panting, diarrhea, tachycardia, pyrexia, pruritus, heart failure in dogs with cardiac disease, exacerbation of adrenal crisis in dogs with hypoadrenocorticism
Testosterone		0.5-1 mg/kg (up to a maximal dose of 30 mg) q 24 h orally (D, C)		Aggressive behavior, greasy haircoat, prostatic hypertrophy, hepatotoxicity
Estrogen		0.02 mg/kg q 48 h for 6-12 wk orally or q 24 h for 3 wk, then 1 wk off, then repeat cycle (D).	Estrogen-responsive dermatosis	Estrus induction, bone marrow suppression, hepatotoxicity, pyometra, spontaneous abortion
Melatonin		3-6 mg q 12-24 h for 2-3 mo (D)	Cyclic follicular dysplasia, follicular dysplasia, alopecia.	Abscess formation with injection of repository capsules.
Growth hormone*		0.1 IU/kg q 56 h for 6 wk (D)	Adrenal sex hormone imbalance, growth-hormone responsive disease (I do not recommend treatment with this drug).	Anaphylaxis, acromegaly, diabetes mellitus

Appendices

A. Breed Predilections

Abyssinian cat	Ceruminous otitis externa Psychogenic alopecia
Airedale	Adult-onset demodicosis
Akita	Pemphigus foliaceus Sebaceous adenitis Uveodermatologic syndrome
Basset Hound	Atopy Intertrigo Malassezia dermatitis Seborrhea
Beagle	Atopy Demodicosis IgA deficiency
Belgian Tervuren	Vitiligo
Border Collie	Systemic lupus erythematosus
Borzoi	Hypothyroidism
Boston Terrier	Atopy Demodicosis Intertrigo
Boxer	Atopy Cyclic follicular dysplasia Demodicosis Hyperadrenocorticism Muzzle and/or pedal bacterial furunculosis
Bullmastiff	Bacterial furunculosis
Bullterrier	Atopy Acrodermatitis Bacterial furunculosis Solar dermatitis
Cairn Terrier	Atopy
Chesapeake Bay Retriever	Atopy
Chihuahua	Demodicosis
Chow Chow	Adrenal sex hormone abnormalities Pemphigus foliaceus Demodicosis Hyposomatotropism Hypothyroidism
Collie	Dermatomyositis

	Lupus erythematosus
	Pemphigus erythematosus
Curly-coated Retriever	Follicular dysplasia
Dachshund	Bacterial pyoderma
	Color dilution alopecia
	Hyperadrenocorticism
	Hypothyroidism
	Juvenile cellulitis
	Malassezia dermatitis
	Pattern alopecia
	Pinnal vasculitis
	Sterile pyogranulomatous dermatitis
	Sterile nodular panniculitis
Dalmatian	Atopy
	Demodicosis
	Solar dermatitis
Doberman	Acral lick dermatitis
	Bacterial pyoderma
	Color dilution alopecia
	Demodicosis
	Drug reaction (particularly against sulfonamides)
	Follicular dysplasia
	Hypothyroidism
	Vitiligo
English Bulldog	Atopy
	Bacterial pyoderma
	Cyclic follicular dysplasia
	Demodicosis
	Intertrigo
	Hypothyroidism
	Malassezia dermatitis
	Sterile pyogranuloma syndrome
German Shepherd	Atopy
	Bacterial pyoderma
	Ear tip fly dermatitis
	Eosinophilic furunculosis
	Flea-bite hypersensitivity
	Food adverse reaction
	Idiopathic onychomadesis
	Mucocutaneous bacterial pyoderma
	Pemphigus erythematosus
	Pituitary dwarfism
	Systemic lupus erythematosus
	Tarsal fistulae
	Vitiligo
Golden Retriever	Acral lick dermatitis
	Atopy
	Bacterial pyoderma
	Hypothyroidism
	Juvenile cellulitis
	Nasal hypopigmentation ("Dudley nose")
	Pyotraumatic dermatitis

Gordon Setter	Atopy Hypothyroidism
Great Dane	Acral lick dermatitis Bacterial pyoderma Callus formation Demodicosis Hypothyroidism
Great Pyrenees	Demodicosis Pyotraumatic dermatitis
Irish Setter	Atopy Color dilution alopecia Hypothyroidism
Irish Water Spaniel	Follicular dysplasia
Jack Russel Terrier	Atopy Demodicosis
Keeshond	Alopecia X due to sex hormone imbalances Hyposomatotropism Hypothyroidism
Labrador Retriever	Acral lick dermatitis Atopy Bacterial pyoderma Food adverse reaction Pyotraumatic dermatitis Seborrhea
Lhasa Apso	Atopy Malassezia dermatitis
Malamute	Zinc-responsive dermatitis
Newfoundland	Bacterial pyoderma Pyotraumatic dermatitis
Old English Sheepdog	Atopy Demodicosis
Pekingese	Intertrigo
Persian Cat	Cheyletiellosis Dermatophytosis Intertrigo Seborrhea
Pointer	Acral mutilation Demodicosis Hereditary lupoid dermatosis
Pomeranian	Adrenal sex hormone abnormalities Hyposomatotropism
Poodle	Hyperadrenocorticism Hypothyroidism Injection reactions Sebaceous adenitis (Standard)
Portuguese Water Dog	Follicular dysplasia

Pug	Atopy
	Intertrigo
Rhodesian Ridgeback	Dermoid sinus
Rottweiler	Bacterial pyoderma
	Vasculitis
	Vitiligo
Samoyed	Sebaceous adenitis
Schipperke	Pemphigus foliaceus
Scottish Terrier	Atopy
Shar-pei	Atopy
	Bacterial pyoderma
	Demodicosis
	Food adverse reaction
	Hypothyroidism
	IgA deficiency
	Intertrigo
	Mucinosis
Schnauzer	Atopy
	Aurotrichia
	Hypothyroidism
	Schnauzer comedo syndrome
	Superficial suppurative necrolytic Dermatitis
Shetland Sheepdog	Dermatomyositis
	Lupus erythematosus
Shi-Tzu	Atopy
Siamese Cat	Food adverse reaction
	Hypotrichosis
	Periocular leukotrichia
	Vitiligo
Siberian Husky	Eosinophilic furunculosis
	Follicular dysplasia
	Zinc-responsive dermatitis
	Atopy
Spaniels	Food adverse reaction
	Hypothyroidism
	Idiopathic onychomadesis
	Intertrigo
	Malassezia dermatitis
	Psoriasiform-lichenoid dermatosis (English Springer Spaniel)
	Seborrhea
St. Bernard	Acral lick dermatitis
	Bacterial pyoderma
Viszla	Sebaceous adenitis
Weimaraner	Sterile pyogranulomatous syndrome

West Highland White Terrier	Atopy
	Food adverse reaction
	Malassezia dermatitis
	Seborrhea
Yorkshire Terrier	Color dilution alopecia
	Injection reactions
	Traction alopecia

B. Questionnaire

What is the main problem? _____

At what age was this condition first noticed? _____

Has there ever been any previous dermatitis? □ Yes □ No

Do the symptoms vary?

If the dermatitis has been present for some time are the symptoms worse in:

□ spring? □ summer? □ autumn? □ winter?

Are the symptoms present all year round? □ Yes □ No

If yes, would there be a time of no symptoms at some stage? □ Yes □ No

What (if anything) causes a worsening of symptoms? _____

What helps? _____

Home details:

Do you have any other pets – and if so how many?

__cats __dogs __birds __other

Do you know of any relative of this pet that has skin problems?

□ Yes □ No

Does any human in the house have skin problems? □ Yes □ No

Where does this pet sleep? _____

Have there been any other illnesses? _____

Bathing and fleas:

Does bathing: □ help □ worsen □ make no difference

How often do you prefer to bath your pet? □ weekly □ monthly □ rarely

When was the last time a flea was seen on this pet? ____ other pets? ____

What is the current flea treatment on this pet? _____

Is flea treatment used on other pets? _____

Medication:

If previous medications have been used, do you know what they were?

□ Yes □ No

If yes, were they: □ shampoos □ rinses □ injections □ tablets □ ointments

Last tablet given (date): _____ Response: □ none □ some □ good

Last injection given: (date): _____ Response: □ none □ some □ good

Is your dog on heartworm tablets? □ No □ Yes: □ daily □ monthly

Diet:

What do you normally feed your pet? □ cans □ dry □ table scraps □ meat

If meat – which types? _____

Any other foods? (eg., vitamins, toast, biscuits) _____

Have you ever fed a special diet? □ No □ Yes: What? _____

_____

Symptoms?

Have any of the following been observed?

□ sores □ scabs □ dandruff □ hair loss □ odor □ hives □ redness

□ sweating □ ear problems □ watery eyes □ heat □ weight loss

□ weight gain □ vomiting □ diarrhea □ tiredness □ depression

□ increased appetite □ increased thirst

Does your pet:

□ rub at the face □ lick or chew the paws □ scratch at the sides

□ roll on the back □ bite at the tail area □ lick the stomach area

□ sneeze □ snort □ wheeze other? _____

What do you think could be the cause of the problem? _____

_____

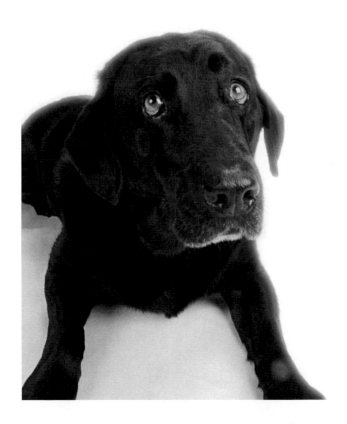

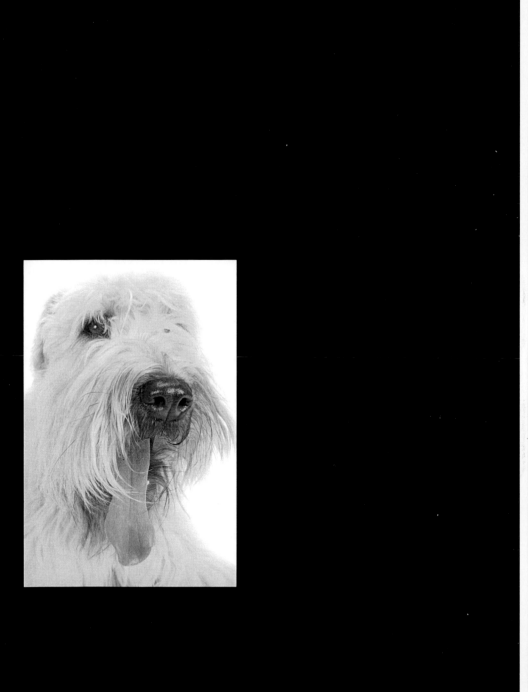

Recommended Readings

Bonagura JD. Ed. *Kirk's Current Veterinary Therapy (XII and XIII)*. Philadelphia, WB Saunders, 1995 and 2000.

Campbell KL. Ed. *The Veterinary Clinics of North America-Small Animal Practice: Dermatology, Vol. 29 (6)*. Philadelphia, WB Saunders, 1995.

Feldman EC, Nelson RW. *Canine and Feline Endocrinology and Reproduction*. 2nd Ed. Philadelphia, WB Saunders, 1996.

Greene CE. *Infectious Diseases of the Dog and Cat*. 2nd Ed. Philadelphia, WB Saunders, 1998.

Griffen CE, Kwochka KW, MacDonald JM. Eds. *Current Veterinary Dermatology*. St. Louis, Mosby, 1993.

Kunkle G. Ed. *The Veterinary Clinics of North America-Small Animal Practice: Feline Dermatology, Vol. 25 (4)*. Philadelphia, WB Saunders, 1995.

Kwochka KW, Willemse T, von Tscharner C. Eds. *Advances in Veterinary Dermatology, Volume 3*. Oxford, Butterworth Heinemann, 1998.

Locke PH, Harvey RG, Mason IS. *Handbook of Small Animal Dermatology*. Oxford, Pergamon, 1995.

Moriello KA, Mason IS. *Canine and Feline Endocrinology and Reproduction*. 2nd Ed. Philadelphia, WB Saunders, 1996.

Ogilvie GK, Moore AS. *Managing the Veterinary Cancer Patient: A Practice Manual*. Trenton, Veterinary Learning Systems, 1995.

Plumb DC. *Veterinary Drug Handbook*. 3rd Ed. White Bear Lake, Pharma Vet Publishing, 1999.

Reedy RM, Miller WH, Willemse T. *Allergic Skin Diseases of Dogs and Cats*. 2nd Ed. Philadelphia, WB Saunders, 1997.

Scott DW, Miller WH, Griffin CE. *Small Animal Dermatology*. 5th Ed. Philadelphia, WB Saunders, 1995.

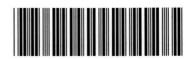